THE
SPICE DIET

THE
SPICE DIET

USE POWERHOUSE FLAVOR TO FIGHT CRAVINGS AND WIN THE WEIGHT-LOSS BATTLE

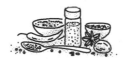

Chef Judson Todd Allen

and Diane Reverand

Foreword by Steve Harvey

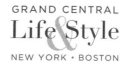

GRAND CENTRAL
Life & Style
NEW YORK • BOSTON

Grand Central Life & Style
Hachette Book Group
1290 Avenue of the Americas, New York, NY 10104
grandcentrallifeandstyle.com
twitter.com/grandcentralpub

First edition: January 2018

Grand Central Life & Style is an imprint of Grand Central Publishing. The Grand Central Life & Style name and logo are trademarks of Hachette Book Group, Inc.

The publisher is not responsible for websites (or their content) that are not owned by the publisher.

The Hachette Speakers Bureau provides a wide range of authors for speaking events. To find out more, go to www.hachettespeakersbureau.com or call (866) 376-6591.

Illustrations copyright © 2018 by Judson Todd Allen

Library of Congress Cataloging-in-Publication Data

Names: Allen, Judson Todd, author. | Reverand, Diane, author.
Title: The spice diet : use powerhouse flavor to fight cravings and win the weight-loss battle / Chef Judson Todd Allen and Diane Reverand ; foreword by Steve Harvey.
Description: First editon. | New York : Grand Central Life & Style, 2018.
Identifiers: LCCN 2017035642| ISBN 9781538727430 (hardback) | ISBN 9781478975090 (audio download) | ISBN 9781538727423 (ebook)
Subjects: LCSH: Weight loss—Popular works. | Cooking (Herbs) | BISAC: HEALTH & FITNESS / Diets. | COOKING / Specific Ingredients / Herbs, Spices, Condiments.
Classification: LCC RM222.2 .A438 2018 | DDC 613.2/5—dc23
LC record available at https://lccn.loc.gov/2017035642

ISBNs: 978-1-5387-2743-0 (hardcover), 978-1-5387-2742-3 (ebook)

Printed in the United States of America

LSC-H

10 9 8 7 6 5 4 3 2 1

I dedicate this book to my family, who I love and cherish so much!

My mom, Joyce Allen, who has been Team Chef Judson from the start and is now my right-hand gal. My grandmother Julia Murray, who is smiling from heaven and, I'm sure, baking up a storm. My brother, Harold Allen, and nephews, Harold, Hayvon, and Javey. And to my sisters and a host of loving and supportive aunts, uncles, and cousins.

I also dedicate this book to one of my greatest heroes and my greatest inspiration for cooking, a man I always set out to emulate, my granddad Judson Murray. At ninety-eight years old, Granddad passed away one week before the The Spice Diet went to print. He was adamant about me turning my dreams into realities, and I know he is smiling from heaven.

One thing I have learned from my weight-loss battle is that in order to release the heavy baggage we carry, discussing our differences and forgiveness is key. One of the biggest tasks for me was to forgive and apologize to my father, Harold Allen. I am thankful to God that I was able to accomplish this before his recent passing in August of 2017. Dad, this book is dedicated to you for being one of my biggest cheerleaders for the book. I know you are enjoying this read from Heaven.

Lastly, I dedicate this book to every person who has struggled with or is currently struggling with an addiction, specifically one that is food related. I encourage you along your journey and am excited for your breakthrough!

CONTENTS

FOREWORD

I am going to be honest with you. I have tried just about every kind of diet around. I have always had trouble with my weight. Over the years, I have learned that "you are what you eat," as the saying goes. If I kept dieting and returning to the foods I loved once I lost the weight, I was beating a dead horse—undermining my efforts. My weight always inched back up. My approach to eating clearly had to change.

When I first moved to Chicago to launch *The Steve Harvey Show*, I needed to get in shape for the television cameras and for my own well-being. I wanted to look fit and to radiate health and energy. I was so determined that I decided to hire a personal chef, along with a nutritionist and trainer to help me change my eating habits, enjoy flavorful, healthy foods, and get me in the best shape. I had heard about Chef Judson Todd Allen, a creative and innovative young chef, who was well-known in Chicago and around the country after his success on *Food Network Star* season 8. The inspirational story of how he cut his weight in half impressed me. He had a degree in food science, which was fascinating. I'd never met a food scientist and was curious how he used science in his cooking. And I heard his food was great!

Chef Judson did not disappoint. His enthusiasm really rubbed off. He prepared three meals a day for me, as well as snacks, and they just kept getting better and better. I don't think he ever served the same dish twice in the first season of my show. In fact, I lost ten pounds in three weeks without ever feeling like I was dieting. I went on to lose more than thirty pounds. Losing the weight was not a struggle. The food was so delicious, I never felt I was missing out on anything. He helped me to transform the way I thought about food.

I learned so much from him. Being able to make a lifetime commitment to healthy eating depended on getting to the root of my issues with food.

He showed me how to "cheat" on my favorite foods by substituting healthy ingredients and spice combinations without sacrificing any of the flavor or texture. He was a stickler for portion control. After a while, I didn't notice that I was eating less, because my food was so delicious and satisfying.

A few outstanding dishes left a lasting impression on me. His Special "Fried" Chicken, which was organic chicken marinated in a crazy blend of spices and crusted with pecans and fresh parsley, looked just like pieces of dark golden fried chicken, but it was baked in the oven in a healthy way. I also appreciated his creativity when he made a healthier version of cornbread, one of my favorites, by using cauliflower, jalapeño, and other ingredients for a comparable yet brand-new experience that was totally satisfying. Given my long days, I really appreciated the snacks, especially his health bars. One of my favorites was his Nut Berry Maple Bourbon Bar, which was loaded with healthy ingredients and packed with protein. Just wait until you try 'em. You will fall in love with these bars! The recipes are all in *The Spice Diet*.

Pay attention to what my friend Chef Judson says. I am so glad he is sharing his unique food sense and mouth-watering recipes so that all of you can benefit as I did. He is a food genius and a brilliant coach. He will help you to transform your relationship with food. Say good-bye to food cravings! As an added bonus, you'll become a first-rate home cook while you are losing weight. Enjoy the delicious, healthy food that Chef Judson serves up. I think it's pretty clear just how proud I am of Chef Judson conquering one of the hardest things so many of us deal with: weight issues. My hope is that *The Spice Diet* will not only wake up your taste buds, but also change your life for the long haul. You have never been on a "diet" like this before.

—Steve Harvey, October, 2017

A NOTE FROM A FORMERLY "HEAVYWEIGHT" CHEF

Before I created the Spice Diet, I lived in a state of diet distress—360 pounds of distress!—for more than twenty years. I thought the foods I craved and the foods I should eat were totally different. I would swear off all the bad stuff cold turkey and go all in. Disciplined for a while, I ate sad, minuscule portions of bland fare, or sometimes nothing at all. When I lost a pound or two, I celebrated by "cheating" with indulgent, unhealthy foods. That one slice of pizza I promised myself as a reward became the entire pie. I was left feeling defeated and disgusted afterward.

To get back on track, I would punish myself with an austere regimen, and the cycle would start all over again. I learned firsthand that the feast-or-famine dynamic is hard on the body and harder on the spirit. It's the perfect recipe for packing on pounds, falling into a world of depression, and living a disappointing life.

I knew my love of food was at the heart of my problem and realized it had to be part of the solution, so I made some smart choices. During my college years, I studied food science and human nutrition to learn the science of flavors and how to work with food in a healthy way. As I studied what I needed to know about the science of food, my weight continued to escalate. When I developed borderline hypertension and high cholesterol, coupled with depression and self-hatred, I knew it was time to put what I was learning into action. I had my whole life in front of me, but my addiction to food had me on a deadly course. There was no question that I had to change.

This "do or die" realization led me to develop the spice diet. From my college coursework and personal experience, I knew that restrictive fad diets weren't going to cut it. Flavor was the key to success. I knew I could reduce my portions if what I was supposed to eat tasted great. I realized that the way to win my lifelong struggle with my weight was by using spices—a powerful source of flavor.

I love food so much that becoming a chef was a calling. Food is such an integral part of my life that I still dream about it to this day. After college, I went on to study at Le Cordon Bleu in Paris and traveled around Europe studying and experiencing food to refine my cooking skills. In that time, I managed to lose more than 160 pounds and reversed my hypertension and high cholesterol by changing the way I ate. Through my transformation, I learned to love me, and hard!! I have worked with food ever since and have kept the weight off for more than ten years.

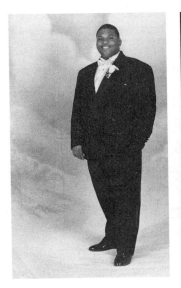 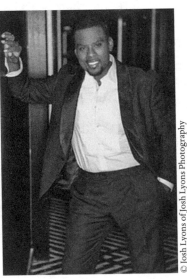

© Josh Lyons of Josh Lyons Photography

Once I felt better in my own body and confident that I could overcome my food addiction for the long term, I developed *The Spice Diet*. My purpose is to teach what I have learned to the millions who struggle with weight issues, to help them to heal their minds, bodies, and spirits through food. I am sharing my program in the hopes that you will lose weight, boost your energy, and develop a renewed spirit and great health.

The Spice Diet dismantles and redefines the word *diet*, a four-letter word with a whole lot of baggage. I'm so over the D-word being synonymous with deprivation and self-loathing. A diet is a habit—nothing more. Habits can become a lifestyle you control or an addiction that controls you. Because you are going to eat every day for the rest of your life, you already have a diet. Right now, it just may not be a healthy diet. *The Spice Diet* is the way to break free from your destructive behavior patterns, so that you can live the life you want and have only imagined—until now.

If you give me thirty days, I promise to get you a healthier and leaner body and make you a great home cook at the same time. I know it's a big promise. I am confident in my plan, because I, along with hundreds of others, am living proof that it works.

—*Chef Judson Todd Allen, April 2017*

INTRODUCTION
Heaven for Food Lovers

Using the principles of food science, I am offering you a plan for eating that seems lavish and self-indulgent, all while satisfying your food cravings *and* reducing your appetite in a healthy way. *The Spice Diet* will help you to break your addiction to unhealthy foods without feeling deprived. My way of eating delivers the flavors you love without the salt, unhealthy fats, and processed carbohydrates that defeat your best efforts to lose weight while they destroy your health.

I've found that one of the greatest challenges for people trying to eat and live well is how to breathe life into their cooking. I hear it all the time: "I get so bored eating healthy, because everything begins to taste the same," or better yet, "I just stick to my salt, garlic seasoning, and black pepper because I have absolutely no idea how to use all those other spices." My goal is to inspire you to get into the kitchen to prepare irresistible, healthy meals. I want you to learn to eat food that supports your health and well-being, instead of being your downfall.

My practical program delivers rapid weight loss—usually ten pounds in a month—by using flavor to satisfy your taste buds and ultimately changing the way you think, feel, and approach healthy foods. In most kitchens, spice racks are used as kitchen decor, not as a functional part of everyday cooking. Those pretty glass jars often have never been touched, and the spices are stale and too old to use—at least that was true in my mother's kitchen. Sorry, Mom.

I want to teach you to use individual spices, spice blends, and natural ingredient combinations that are nutritionally healing to the body. These taste enhancers range from simple, pure flavors to fusion cuisine like

Korean-Latin mash-ups. Adding layers of flavor to your food involves using imagination along with practical techniques to build delicious, healthy meals. *The Spice Diet* will teach you how to create customized flavor profiles that reduce your food cravings by retraining your taste buds. I want my approach to food to inspire you to fall in love, or fall back in love, with your kitchen. You will enjoy a new relationship with your favorite foods, now prepared in a wholesome, palate-pleasing way.

After I tell the story of my own transformation, I will share with you the heart of my program: everything you need to know about herbs and spices, including their flavor characteristics, so you can incorporate them into your cooking to reduce your cravings and heal your body. My recipes deliver powerhouse flavor, and at the same time, my spice blends are functional. The spices I use are medically proven to lower blood sugar, reduce inflammation, settle your digestive system, and more. These delicious blends work with your system from the inside, improving your health, boosting your metabolism, and promoting weight loss. "Fire Up" sidebars throughout the book describe how specific spices can help you lose weight.

In chapter 3, I take a hard look at food addictions and cravings. Understanding what happens in your brain that drives you to overeat should make it clear to you that being overweight is not simply a matter of willpower. I will take a look at obesity in this country and the toll that weighing more than you should takes on your health. My goal is to make you hyperaware of the health risks associated with being overweight and show you how little weight you have to lose to influence your health for the better.

To begin to make healthy eating a habit, you have to create a weight loss mind-set. You have to believe you can do it and make a serious commitment. You have to face your truths head on by addressing the issues that got you where you are with your weight. I'll give you advice on how to break up with your current relationship with food, which obviously isn't working. I will show you how to make the shift to mindful eating. I will cover not only the psychological and spiritual aspects of weight problems, but will also present practical information, including the nitty-gritty on processed foods, portion control, and getting more movement into your life. Adam Zickerman, the founder of InForm Fitness and the author of the *New York Times* bestseller *Power of 10*, has created two fifteen-minute resistance band workouts for *The Spice Diet* that you only have to do twice a week. Once you have covered this material, you are ready to roll up your sleeves and jump right in for the first thirty days of taking control of what you eat, a month that will change your life.

The Spice Diet has two phases:

- **Phase 1** is when significant change happens. You will form healthy habits, and your confidence preparing home-cooked meals using spice blends will grow. This phase lasts thirty days, during which most people lose at least ten pounds. If your goal is to lose additional weight, you can stick with Phase 1 until you are close to your dream weight.
- **Phase 2** is when you perfect the healthy habits you began to develop in Phase 1, maintain your weight loss, and transition to your new dietary lifestyle—for the rest of your life. You can continue to lose weight gradually during Phase 2, but the more rapid results of Phase 1 are always there for you if you want to return to it at any time.

There are two weeks of meal plans for each stage to give you an idea of how well you will be eating for breakfast, lunch, dinner, dessert, and snacks. I have created mouth-watering recipes for Phases 1 and 2, including a "Peach Cobbler" Power Bar and a Citrus Protein Bar, which you can make yourself. These powerhouse flavor recipes will prove to you that *The Spice Diet* is anything but boring. Imagine eating a Guiltless Lemon-Blueberry Cake Milk Shake, South-of-the-Border Grilled Corn Bisque, Honey-Lemon Baked Chicken, and Sweet Potato Crumble as you steadily lose weight!

The recipes are followed by twenty-five spice blends I have built, including N'awlins Spiced Pecan Crust Blend, Sour Dill Pickle Blend, and Jamaican Me Crazy Jerk Spice Blend that you can make and keep on hand for an instant flavor boost to just about anything you are preparing. Now you can see what I am getting at: if you are eating food this full of flavor, you will not feel deprived.

Finally, I want to provide you with lifetime strategies that will help you keep the weight off, like how to avoid losing your resolve when you eat out, on special occasions, and on vacation. I offer advice on how to get through the holidays without gaining weight. No one is perfect. It helps to have strategies to resist temptations.

I'm not promising that this will be easy, but if you're willing to put in the work and dedication to change now and keep it going, the spice blends and ingredients in my recipes—and the ones you will learn to create—will propel you toward your goal. It's time to fight and be the master of your fate. Put the power of spices to work for you. My plan won't only change the number on your scale or the size of your clothes. *The Spice Diet* will change your life!

1

PORTRAIT OF A FOOD ADDICT

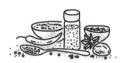

Years ago, when I was in high school, a couple of my so-called friends got their hands on my medical report from a recent physical exam. They high lighted my weight and the words "morbidly obese." They passed out copies to what felt like everyone in the school. People stared at me, laughing, and poked each other when I walked by. Some made comments under their breath. Others came right out and called me names that are still painful to repeat. See, it wasn't just the fact that they were laughing and judging me; it was also the realization that they all knew the one thing I hated most about myself. The incident at school made me ashamed. I felt grotesque in the eyes of other people.

As a teenager, I considered myself "thick" or overweight. I knew I weighed more than was normal for my height, age, and sex, but that had been true since I was a child. I learned the hard way that there is a big difference between being overweight and being obese. I was sixteen years old when I discovered the true meaning of the term *morbidly obese*. Technically, obesity is a number on a table of data and is known to cause many diseases, but I experienced firsthand that being obese was doing more than compromising my health. I was in shock to find out that I was suffering from obesity at such a young age. Obesity is considered a disease marked by excessive storage of body fat and a body mass index (BMI) over 30. I was embarrassed beyond belief. I cannot tell you how hard I was on myself. My self-loathing was overwhelming.

You would think this humiliating experience would make me change the way I ate, but unfortunately, my cycles between healthy and destructive behavior only got worse. When life got too stressful, my emotions would take over. I would binge eat and build more barriers between myself and the rest of the world. This had been my pattern since I was a child.

Everyone in my immediate family was overweight. My father and brother were athletic and didn't let their weight get totally out of control, but my mother and I always struggled. I was heavy from the start. The men in my family could really throw down. My grandfather, who is from Louisiana, prepared rich, decadent comfort food. I can still smell his seafood gumbo and rice, fried catfish coated with cornmeal—shaken in a brown bag, of course—with a side of creamy grits, and his famous barbecue ribs. My dad always got me with his sinfully rich and creamy potato salad and savory yet sweet spaghetti. Every meal was flat-out delicious. I'm talking about the type of food that makes your eyes roll to the back of your head and requires a couch and a two- to ten-hour nap afterward.

My mother's cooking was another story. Busy working as a teacher, she was efficient about preparing meals. I am sure by now you know where this is going. She had a weekly rotation of seven dinners she repeated each week. They were square meals, meant to be healthy, but they were pretty boring. My brother and I either indulged at our grandparents' house or ate fast food. Although Mom is definitely going to chase me with a broom after this, she, too, can admit that she depended heavily on fast food and restaurants to please us all.

There was always junk food in the house. My mother shopped at big box stores and bought everything jumbo size. I had an insatiable hunger. I remember making pantry raids like it was yesterday. She would buy a big canister of nacho cheese and an outrageously large bag of tortilla chips, which I would devour in the middle of the night as if I were in a trance. I ate stacks of PB&J sandwiches on white bread and huge bowls of salty popcorn dripping with melted butter.

Ever since grade school, I was one of the biggest kids in the class. Every time I moved up a grade, I looked around to check out if there were others who were bigger or the same size as I was. If there were others kids who were as heavy, I was relieved, because the ridicule would be shared. I wouldn't be the sole object of my classmates' teasing.

My parents divorced when I was very young, and though I always knew my dad loved me, deep down inside I felt he was hard on me and that there was a bit of a disconnect. He wanted the best for me, but I felt I didn't measure up to his expectations. My older brother, who was always in some type of trouble, looked like my dad and was a "macho" athlete like him. I wasn't as athletic. OK, I will keep this completely honest: Other than swimming, I was not really into sports. I was a go-getter, ambitious, and a great student always earning excellent grades. I guess being smart and somewhat sensitive at times, I was an easy target for the incessant reminders of all my shortcomings. My father constantly told me I was getting heavy and never hesitated to comment on the ups and downs of my weight. He pressed me to lose some pounds. Now I understand that he just wanted to make my life better, but then I only saw it as criticism, and my self-esteem plummeted even further.

My mother took me to shop in the husky clothes section, where the choice was limited to elastic-waist pants. For my eighth-grade graduation, my dad had to take me suit shopping at the Big & Tall store. Rather than the malls and department stores where my friends shopped, Big & Tall became my destination.

I wanted to be stylish. I was a skinny person in a fat person's body. As I got older and made my own choices, I bought clothes that were too small—2X instead of 4X—which only accentuated my weight problem. I always did manage to create a well-put-together look. The sky was the limit when it came to my haircuts and shoes.

I was in denial about how overweight I was. I, like many, hit a point in my weight struggles and self-image when I became completely blinded to the reality of my situation. When I looked in the mirror, I rarely saw my overweight self. My mom and dad would remind me that when I was ten years old, I always went straight for the rack of clothes that did not fit.

When I was young and bullied because of my weight, I used two coping mechanisms to handle it: humor and food. After my braces were removed in the fifth grade, I had a bright, white smile, which I used to deflect ridicule. I developed a big personality, which wasn't easy, given my weight-consciousness. I created a bigger-than-life alter ego who loved being the center of attention. I was funny and charismatic, the life of the party. No one knew the real me inside. I protected myself and covered up my self-hate by entertaining and pleasing people. At school, I could laugh off the jokes made at my expense and make other people laugh along with me.

I wasn't very social outside of school. I spent a lot of time at home feeling lonely and disconnected. I created a retreat for myself in our basement where I became a prisoner of my appetite. It was a cold, unfinished basement with support poles spaced regularly throughout. The concrete floor was covered with tiles. I had an area rug to define my sanctuary space, an old, cushy gold velvet chair, and a TV with cable and VHS and DVD players. My brother's improvised gym, consisting of some mats and improvised weights, was on the other side of the basement, not that I was ever tempted to work out there. I went to binge in the privacy of my basement screening room, away from the disapproving eyes of my mother. My weekend regimen was to confine myself to my domain in the basement and lounge in my comfy chair, watching a good movie and binging on greasy bagged food, soda, chips, and candy bars to soothe my battered psyche.

In grammar school, between fourth and eighth grade, I frequently went to the corner store that was also a hole-in-the-wall greasy spoon, where I ordered fries, pizza puffs, and gyros. My portions were way out of control. Mexican food was another vice. My meal of choice was the steak burrito with extra meat, cheese, and sour cream. If I felt the added extras were skimpy, I would politely ask for more. I would eat two days' worth of food in one sitting. The store packed all the food I ordered in one bag along with a two-liter bottle of soda. I would sneak into the house with my stash and go straight to the basement. I could never eat enough to fill me up.

My parents wanted me to do well in school, so I never had an after-school job. When my mother gave me money, I saved it and eventually used it for my trips to the corner store. I got good at getting money from her. I'd say, "Mom, I'm going to the store—need anything? A bag of chips? An Almond Joy?" I knew she'd want something. I'd always use the change to get more food for myself, which I devoured alone in the basement. A "grammar school conman," I would manipulate my mother to feed my food addiction. Not only did I hurt myself, but I also undermined my mother's efforts to lose weight.

She noticed how big I was getting and started to go through the trash. She knew I wasn't getting fat on the food she was cooking. When she realized what I was doing, she tried to restrict me. I outsmarted her by hiding my trash at the bottom of the garbage can. I didn't think about it at the time, but pawing through the garbage to bury the evidence of my bingeing was definitely not normal. My compulsion to eat was making me do crazy things to cover up something that I knew was wrong.

By eighth grade, I weighed more than two hundred pounds.

I could tell you story after story about gorging myself on nachos, making fast-food runs at all hours, and other tales of my poor food choices. I was never satisfied, because I wasn't nourishing my body. I was only filling it with processed, unhealthy garbage that always left me wanting more.

My mother was worried about me, especially as I was approaching high school. She was a yo-yo dieter. She had gained weight during pregnancy and had difficulty managing her weight after my brother and I were born. Trying every fad diet, she would eat next to nothing. She lost weight when she followed restrictive eating plans. But as soon as she went off these diets, she regained the weight she had lost and more.

She was so compassionate. She told me everything she had been through, and the sense of failure she felt when she couldn't control her eating. She knew what my weight was costing me. She wanted me to be happy more than anything. She started a campaign to get me to stop eating junk food. I'd come home from school and say how hungry I was. She'd respond, "Have an apple. It will hold you over until dinner. We're having chili." I wanted McDonald's—right then. I'd get angry if I couldn't eat what I wanted when I wanted it, which was all the time. I was like an alcoholic or drug addict in withdrawal.

As a last resort, my mother put a lock on the refrigerator door. A lock couldn't stop me. I still made runs to the greasy spoon on the corner for the food that had become like crack to me. The food and this destructive lifestyle had a stranglehold on me.

She was also responsible for one of the most mortifying experiences I've ever had. She made me go with her to her weight-loss group meeting. There I was, a fat, cranky adolescent boy, in a room full of overweight women. Those kinds of programs work for some people, but I didn't connect to what they were saying in any way. I looked at the leaders of the group and knew they had not struggled with their weight the way I was struggling. I saw thin people preaching that skinless chicken and steamed broccoli were the answer. To my mind, they had no idea what it was like to be addicted to food. I was hostile and wanted them to get out of my face.

Feeling completely out of place with all those women, all I could think of, with horror, was, "What if someone I know sees me here?"

Things changed when I started high school. I had more freedom and could do what I wanted. Since I was self-conscious about being fat, I didn't want people to see me eating. I'd go the whole school day without food. Skipping lunch in the cafeteria wasn't hard. The food was nasty and disgusting. But I thought about food all day. When school ended at two thirty or three, I would take the bus to Wendy's for a Frosty and two Double Stacks. Then I would return home to snack until dinner.

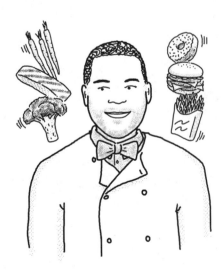

At sixteen, I started driving my family's extra, old car to school. In the morning, I'd stop at Burger King and inhale two croissant breakfast sandwiches and a large OJ. I wouldn't eat lunch. After school, I'd go to a restaurant with friends. I was self-conscious about what I ordered with them, and I never allowed myself to pig out in the company of others. I might have an order of wings and fries—no more than what anyone else was eating. No one had any idea what I did in the privacy of my binge cave.

I managed to lose weight a number of times during high school. I starved myself and worked out endlessly. I was never thin, but I did lose weight. Then my addiction would kick in. It was hard to pass a fast-food restaurant without stopping. I promised myself I would just have a taste, but I couldn't restrain myself. I was hooked.

During my senior year of high school, I decided that since I couldn't live without food, I had to find a way to live making food the center of my life without having to be addicted to it. It was then that I decided to study food science and human nutrition at the University of Illinois at Urbana-Champaign, to learn how to approach food in a healthy way. It was one of the best decisions I've ever made.

With all the best intentions and hope that food science and nutrition would be the answer to my weight loss prayers, my weight continued to escalate during my college years. I was doing well and had tons of friends, but I still couldn't control my eating. Although I was determined to change, it took no time for me to be tempted again. While some students gain the classic "freshman fifteen," I gained more than sixty pounds my freshman year. From buffet style meals to deep-dish pizzas at friends' homes to late-night food runs after partying, I found myself bigger than ever before.

Then my weight began to affect my health. I developed borderline hypertension and high cholesterol. My addiction to food was already damaging me. There are size 4 people who diet just to fit in a size 2 swimsuit, but for me, the stakes had become much higher. I wanted desperately to change.

I longed to have sex appeal. I needed to attract attention beyond "He's cute for a fat boy," "He's like a brother to me," and, my favorite, "He makes me laugh, but he's not my type." My need to lose weight was more urgent once my health became compromised. If I remained obese, I was writing my own ticket to an early grave.

Even with this awareness, it took a visual to jolt me to change. I received a photograph of myself in the mail, which had been taken on the day I graduated from college. I had just received my degree in food science. The elated expression on my face said I was ready to take on the world, but the image before my eyes said something else. I was shocked by how I looked. At 5 feet 9 inches, I weighed more than 360 pounds, about twice my ideal weight according to medical charts. Somehow that photo caught what I had been denying for a long time. I felt as if someone had punched me in the gut.

"Why didn't anyone tell me I'd gotten so big?" were the first words out of my mouth.

The truth was, people who loved me had tried to tell me in all kinds of ways and had been doing so for a long time. I didn't want to hear it. Although it was fine for me to be down on myself, I was too sensitive to take criticism from anyone else, to admit what a big problem I had.

Holding that picture in my hand, I came to my senses. I realized I would never be able to change without facing the roots of my addiction to food. The struggle, pain, self-loathing, rejection, and family issues from childhood still resonated inside me. For the first time in my life, I knew I had to drop the facade I had so carefully constructed. I had to allow myself to be vulnerable if I ever was to break out of the prison of my addiction. As much as I wanted to lose weight, I had never been able to stop stuffing down my dark, agonizing feelings with food for the long term. I had to face my demons so that the real me could emerge from the armor of alienation my addiction had created. I was determined to take control of my eating, my health, and my life.

That day, when I finally realized that enough was enough, I put my education to work—for my own benefit. I had all the pieces of the puzzle: I just had to put them together. I knew the chemistry of how ingredients work together. I had learned the psychology of sensory analysis. I was prepared with techniques that I could use to achieve the flavors I wanted. Having studied nutrition, I was ready to nourish my body properly for the first time in my adult life.

I'm proud of what I have been able to achieve, but I am here to tell you that the pull to relapse never really goes away. I have armed myself with strategies that allow me to indulge my food cravings now and then without going over the top. Although I've kept my weight down, I am still not where

I want to be. I continue to envision myself with six-pack abs, and I am working toward that goal.

When you can look back and see how far you have come, discipline becomes habitual. Just as you relied on bad eating habits to comfort you in the past, you will turn to nourishing, high-energy, flavorful food to satisfy your hunger and restore you to robust health and well-being. And, as a bonus, you will learn to make magic in the kitchen. I want *The Spice Diet* to do for you what it has done for me. Give it a try. You won't look back.

2

THE ARCHITECT OF FLAVOR

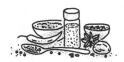

Ten years after I seriously committed to becoming a "smaller" person, I was in Nashville, Tennessee, to work on a consulting project. The day before an important meeting, I received an unexpected call from Steve Harvey himself. I discovered later that my marketing and operations director knew a member of Steve Harvey's personal team and had shared my background and contact information with him in the hopes that he would in turn pass it along to Steve. Steve had recently made a national announcement that he was going to launch a TV show in Chicago, my stomping grounds, and was in search of a personal chef.

I was shocked to hear his voice on the phone. After I stammered a greeting, he said, "Hey, Chef, I hear you are the healthy flavor chef. I want you to meet me at the NBC studio at 5:00 a.m. tomorrow with a packaged breakfast, lunch, and dinner. I will see you then."

I was speechless, but managed to say I'd be there. He had presented me with a once-in-a-lifetime opportunity. I had to go into strategy mode. I was four hundred miles away from Chicago and needed to figure out how to prepare a full day's worth of meals for him and have them ready and delivered by dawn the next morning. Of course, I consulted with the Man Upstairs and my family for advice on how I should proceed.

I made my apologies and rescheduled my big meeting. I took the first flight out of Nashville that evening. When I got to Chicago, I had to find a twenty-four-hour grocery store that offered quality, fresh products, then prepare and package the meals. That morning, I was a firecracker, extremely nervous, but I had my game face on and was ready to present as the sun came up! All I could think was, "Jud, you are not going to squander this opportunity. Now serve it."

MY AUDITION MENU FOR STEVE HARVEY

Breakfast: Honey Caramelized Pear and Fig Fresh Granola and Steel-Cut Oatmeal with Vanilla Almond Milk

Lunch: Roasted Lemon and Chive, Crab-Stuffed Chilean Sea Bass and Wilted Swiss Chard

Dinner: Grilled New Orleans Prawns with Roasted Garlic Quinoa and Sweet Potato Cake

---

I must say, it paid off that I did some preliminary research into the foods Steve loves. Of course, leave it to the "architect of flavor" to take those favorites and make them extraordinary. I dished up some of my proudest culinary creations, including my signature Crab-Stuffed Chilean Sea Bass.

I hit a home run and closed the deal! I became Steve Harvey's personal chef, and he built me a kitchen in his dressing room, which was more like a completely decked-out condo. Steve valued my international culinary studies and was intrigued by my food science degree. In his inimitable voice, he asked, "So I hear you can make healthy food flavorful, huh, and what the hell is a food scientist anyway?" I knew that the Spice Diet would wow him.

He had seen me compete to the finals on season 8 of the Food Network's hit show *Next Food Network Star*. He was impressed that I used that national platform to tell the story of how I struggled and finally overcame my weight problems. We discovered that we had a lot in common. Not only had we both dealt with weight issues, but we also share an insatiable zeal to win. Steve wanted to get in shape for the launch of his television show. During my first few weeks, I worked closely with others on his team, including his nutritionist and personal trainer. After a short amount of time, Steve developed a level of trust in me that spoke to my commitment and character.

I discovered that Steve knows a lot about health, food choices, and exercise. Having researched many weight loss, detox, and general health programs, he has also interviewed countless experts on his radio and television shows. With his opportunity to learn from the top experts, I consider him an expert in the healthy living field—no MD or PhD necessary.

He is one of the most disciplined people I have ever met, which is not hard to believe given his enormous success. Keeping his demanding schedule takes boundless energy. My sous chef and I used my spice and ingredient combinations to design flavor profiles that gave the hardest-working man on TV the energy and health benefits he needed.

Steve loves great-tasting food that has ultimately made him look and feel amazing. One of my proudest moments working for him was when he complimented me on my Lobster Mac and Cheese and Grilled Peach and Kale Salad. He said they were the best he'd ever eaten.

Steve lost ten pounds in three weeks. I helped him achieve these results by managing spices and substituting healthy ingredients into the food he loves. I was able to satisfy his cravings in a nutritious way. He came to terms with his weight struggles with an unwavering commitment to keep the weight off long term by changing his approach to eating. Steve ultimately lost more than thirty pounds. By delivering great nutrition in combination with powerhouse flavors, I helped Steve to change his perception of healthy foods.

I am feeling much better and leaner with your healthy, flavorful food.

—*Steve Harvey*

THE BLISS POINT

When food manufacturers formulate their highly processed food, they aim to set off the pleasure-reward pathways in your brain, the same pathways associated with addiction to drugs and alcohol. I explain this in more detail in the next chapter. The highly palatable foods they produce are designed to make you addicted to their products. The manufacturers are looking for what they have labeled "the bliss point," created by enough sugar, salt, or fat, to make the food irresistible. When I began to take control of my eating, I realized I had to create the bliss point in healthy foods. I had to produce dishes that delivered pure satisfaction. If I could light up the reward center in my brain with food that was good for me, I assumed I would eventually switch my cravings from unhealthy food to healthy food.

I began by weaning myself from the rich, calorie-loaded food that I loved. My first step was to make simple swaps: corn tortillas for flour ones, roasted skinless chicken instead of steak, and plain yogurt instead of sour cream. I switched out cream in recipes, first substituting half-and-half, then whole milk, and then skim milk or light coconut milk. I worked more vegetables into my diet to make up for the bulk I was accustomed to getting from higher-calorie ingredients.

In the old days, I ate mayonnaise straight out of the jar. It was so creamy. I spread it thickly on every sandwich I ate. I even used it in dips. I decided to see if I could swap it out for something creamy with a lower fat content. I made myself a new condiment. I added a little mayonnaise to very good mustard—I especially liked whole-grain mustard for the subtle texture—to make the mustard creamier. It did the trick. The tanginess of the mustard combined with the creaminess of the mayonnaise made this lower-calorie spread my go-to condiment.

As I've mentioned, Mexican food was/is one of my weaknesses. I couldn't get enough sour cream, so I knew I had to come up with a low-fat substitute. I decided to try using plain nonfat yogurt. I know, yogurt is not sour cream, but I had ideas about what to do to amplify the flavor. I added fresh lime juice for acidity, and then I mixed in some fresh herbs to boost the flavor even more. When I took a taste, I loved it. There were endless ways I could change up the herbs to make my new "sour cream" deliciously different each time. It was out with the old, in with the new.

I was infatuated with fried catfish with fries or grits and couldn't get enough of it. I can remember my grandfather taking out the big cast-iron skillet and a can of lard. He would shake the fish in a brown paper bag to coat it with flour, cornmeal, and seasoning. I loved pouring hot sauce and tartar sauce on the crunchy, golden-crusted fish. When I thought about it, it was the crunch—the texture—that I loved.

I decided to reproduce this dish with healthy fat and less salt. I seasoned the fish with Cajun spices and my Chef Blend Hot Sauce, which has the benefit of being very low in sodium, and put the fillets on a baking sheet. For the crust, I combined chopped pecans, lemon zest, parsley, and a small amount of Parmesan cheese just for taste. I brushed the fillet with a little olive oil and then put the nut mixture on top of the fish. Rather than frying the fish, I baked it at a high temperature. The results were just what I wanted. Inside the delicious golden crunch, the fish was moist and tender.

This healthy version was actually better than my grandfather's deep-fried catfish. My taste buds were introduced to flavor that was new and exciting. The crunch was even better than the fried fish. Prepared this way, the fish stimulated my palate. It gave me what I call a total foodgasm! It was a party in my mouth! I had no trouble replacing a deep-fried guilty pleasure with food that was healthy for me.

By experimenting with tasty substitutions and new prep and cooking methods, I was able to scale back and finally to wean myself off food that was making me obese and destroying my health. I came to see that exciting my taste buds with a balance of powerful flavors had the same effect as eating processed food. I was able to find the bliss point again and again. When your brain experiences pleasure from eating wholesome food, your cravings for fast and processed foods diminish.

I promote home-cooked meals for many reasons. When you cook at home, you have complete control over what you are eating. From the quality and freshness of the ingredients you buy to the relative quantity of those ingredients in a dish, from the flavor profile you want to achieve to the method you use to cook the food—there are no restrictions on what you can do in the kitchen. You can create your own bliss point in every meal. I want to give you the tools to become a home cook who is confident about working with food and equipped to make easy meals that do more than satisfy cravings. When you take control of what you eat by preparing your own food, you will have what it takes to get ahead of your weight problems and improve your health.

LAYERING FLAVOR

At a cooking demonstration I was giving a few years ago, a woman in the audience made a comment that I've since made my own. I had been talking about ingredient combinations and building flavor.

She called out, "Chef Judson, you're like an architect!"

Her observation was right on the money. She could not have done a better job of describing what I do with flavor. An architect is not just concerned with the look of a building but the structure and function as well.

The same is true of the Spice Diet. It's about using imagination as well as practical techniques to build delicious, healthy meals. It's based on constructing customized flavor profiles that satisfy your taste buds. The food you eat will look and taste great and will be nourishing and healing at the same time.

Come to think of it, I learned how to build flavor from my family. Nothing made me happier than when my grandfather had a huge pot of chili simmering away on the stove. That wise food lover had a unique way of making flavors pop. The secret ingredients of his chili were malt vinegar, fresh cilantro, and crushed oyster crackers. The acidity from the vinegar, the freshness from the cilantro, and the crunchy texture from the crackers balanced the spicy and rich flavors of the chili. Aromas would waft from the kitchen all day long as he cooked his prized dish slow and low in just the right way. I appreciated what he did and decided to follow in his footsteps. I wanted to construct the food I ate with layers of flavor and texture.

I found that if a recipe or a meal balanced the five flavors—sweet, salty, sour, bitter, and savory—the food was as satisfying as it could get. Incorporating all the flavors wipes out cravings, because you are experiencing all of them. The recipes in chapters 9 and 10 have this layered effect. You'll see— the flavor just keeps coming. I am going to teach you how to create this flavor effect in your own kitchen.

Eating Healthy Never Tasted Like This Before

I have struggled with weight as an adult, blaming my busy lifestyle. It was easier to pick up fast food than to cook. Over time, I developed an insatiable craving for all the wrong foods. Judson introduced me to highly flavored, nutritious meals using spices and ingredient substitutions. Before I experienced his style of food preparation and cooking, I had concluded that "healthy foods" were bland in appearance, tasteless, and generally not very appealing. After tasting the incredible flavor of Judson's cooking, I had no problem adopting a healthier style of eating. Eating healthy never tasted like this before! Consuming high-calorie meals was clearly not necessary for me to feel satisfied. Cooking and eating this way decreased my cravings and put me on the path toward living a healthier lifestyle.

—John W. Lee III

AN ANATOMY OF FLAVOR

Flavor uses all your senses. It has four components: taste, mouthfeel, aroma, and appearance. And then there is the magic: how the food affects your mind and spirit. *Taste* is the effect of the food on your taste buds. *Mouthfeel* is exactly what it sounds like. It involves the sense of touch, such as whether the food is hot or cold; its texture—creamy or crispy; its hotness or sharpness; whether it makes the mouth pucker as a lemon does; and the sound made while it's being eaten. Remember snap, crackle, and pop? That's the sound of crispiness. *Aroma* is responsible for 80 percent or more of the flavor we experience. And let's not forget the *appearance* of your food—our food must always look sexy! Eating engages all your senses as well as inspires an overall feeling of well-being.

If you are going to use spices well, you have to know the properties of the five basic flavors of food: sweet, salty, sour, bitter, and savory, or umami as it is also called. Here is a quick review:

Sweetness brings out the flavors of other ingredients. In chef-speak, that quality is called roundness. Of all the flavors, sweetness requires the greatest amount to register on the taste buds. Sweetness is satiating.

Salt is a flavor enhancer, which is why it is a major ingredient of processed food. It is important in savory dishes. Salt makes you thirsty, which is why pretzels and salty foods are served as finger food at bars. Salt also increases appetite.

Sourness adds brightness to food. From vinegar to lemon juice, sourness contributes acidity to a dish. A sour note is important in savory dishes. Sourness functions to quench thirst. This flavor is refreshing and makes food sparkle.

Bitterness balances sweetness and reduces richness. Your mouth is very sensitive to this cleansing taste. Bitterness is considered stimulating.

Savoriness or **Umami** is known as the "fifth taste profile." The Japanese word *umami* means "pleasant savory taste." This flavor falls between savory and salty. Umami has a meaty taste that makes your mouth feel full. Mushrooms, beef, green tea, shrimp, soybeans, and anchovies are all savory.

You can balance a taste by combining it with its opposite. If you have made something too sweet, add something bitter. If you have been heavy-handed with the salt, add something sour such as lemon juice or vinegar. Opposites balance out each other. I will get into balance in more detail when I discuss creating flavor profiles in chapter 11.

THE DIFFERENCE BETWEEN AN HERB AND A SPICE

I thought I would clear this up once and for all:

A culinary herb is the leaf of a plant. Parsley, sage, and thyme are herbs.

Spices, often dried, come from other parts of the plant, such as the root, stem, bulb, bark, and seeds. For example, cloves are buds; saffron is the stigma of a flower; cinnamon is from the bark; and peppercorns are berries.

SPICE UP YOUR LIFE

In my world, spices don't only come in jars. For me, the word *spice* includes anything that brings out the flavor of food without relying on sodium, refined sugar, processed ingredients, or unhealthy fats. My view of spice goes beyond dried seeds, roots, herbs, and barks. My definition includes taste- and texture-enhancing ingredients such as nuts, berries, edible flowers, and other surprises.

Herbs and spices can add great flavor to foods, but not all of them are delicious alone. Nature created this form of defense to keep animals from eating the plants' leaves. If you have ever accidentally chewed a peppercorn, you know what I'm talking about. The flavors of many herbs and spices are chemical weapons that repel snails, bugs, caterpillars, and other animals and kill germs that could affect the plant. Don't be alarmed. The amount of the chemical in a leaf or seed is a fairly small dose. When you mix herbs and spices with other ingredients, the dose is diluted to just a fraction of its full strength.

Not all herbs and spices cause this reaction. For example, basil, dill, mint, and parsley are delicious on their own. The reason they taste good to us is that their chemical defenses do not have an irritating effect on our mouths. Just think of biting into a mint leaf or topping a juicy tomato with fresh basil.

Scientists have found that herbs and spices that have been grown organically have more flavor because they have higher levels of health-protecting chemicals. Organic herbs and spices are vulnerable to attacks by insects because they are grown without pesticides. When attacked, the organic plants produce more of the aroma and flavor chemicals to repel the insects. If you buy organic herbs and spices, you'll be cooking with fire!

The way you handle herbs can affect their flavor. The defensive chemicals responsible for their flavor can be found in fine, hairlike glands on the surface of the leaves, usually on the underside. This is true of basil, mint, oregano, sage, and thyme. Most other herbs store their flavor chemicals in canals within the leaves. If you crush the herb or cut it very finely, you can damage cells, which release grassy chemicals that can dominate the herb's flavor. You can slow the production of the grassy chemicals by chilling the leaves before you crush or chop them. I will discuss the care and handling of spices and herbs in more detail in chapter 7. I think this little bit of science about the source of the aroma and flavor of herbs and spices is fascinating. I like to know how it all works. No wonder I enjoyed my food science courses at school.

Flavor Families

There are fragrance families for scents, including floral, Oriental, woody, and fresh. These categories of scents, mixed in different combinations and levels of intensity, are used to create perfume. Spices have sensory characteristics as well. To give you an overview of the flavor and aroma profiles of spices, below are fifteen of the most common descriptive labels for spices and the spices that fit into that category.

Bitter: bay leaf, celery seeds, clove, cumin, fenugreek seeds, horseradish, mace, marjoram, savory, Szechuan peppercorns, star anise, turmeric

Cooling: anise, fennel, sweet basil

Earthy: cumin, dried mushrooms, saffron, turmeric

Floral: coriander, lemongrass, saffron, sweet basil, thyme

Fruity: fennel, savory

Herbaceous: dill, oregano, parsley, rosemary, sage, savory, tarragon, thyme

Hot: black pepper, chiles, horseradish, mustard, white pepper

Nutty: black cardamom, coriander seed, cumin seed, fenugreek seeds, mustard seeds, poppy seed, sesame seed

Piney: bay leaf, rosemary, thyme

Pungent: allspice, garlic, ginger, horseradish, marjoram, mustard, onion, paprika, spearmint, star anise

Sour: pomegranate seeds, tamarind

Spicy: bay leaf, cinnamon, clove, coriander, cumin, curry, ginger, marjoram, nutmeg

Sulfurous: chives, garlic, onion

Sweet: allspice, anise, caraway seeds, cinnamon, chervil, clove, dill seed, green cardamom, poppy seed, sesame seed, star anise

Woody: cardamom, Ceylon cinnamon, clove, rosemary, Szechuan peppercorns

If salt and pepper are the full scope of your seasoning repertoire, you might find the number of spices listed here daunting. There is no reason to be intimidated about using spices. I will help you to become comfortable creating powerhouse flavor in your kitchen. This is a completely new territory for you to explore, even if you have experimented a bit. Using spices when you cook will add an exciting dimension to your food. Get ready for a luxury tour of Spice Nation.

Spice Nation

I want to introduce you to the spices you will be using and describe their characteristics. Just as wine experts have a way to talk about wine, there is a special vocabulary for describing the flavors and aromas of spices and herbs. There are five main flavor groups for spices: sweet, pungent, tangy, hot, and amalgamating. Herbs are described as mild, medium, strong, savory, and pungent. I have made a chart that contains common spices and herbs, their flavor groups, and their flavor profiles. An architect of flavor needs to be familiar with the building materials used to construct a balanced, layered harmony of flavors. In order to expand your spice palate, to encourage you to go beyond salt and pepper, you need to have an idea of what a spice will contribute to the overall taste of a dish. Consider this chart Spice 101:

Spices and Herbs

Allspice	Sweet	Warm and sweetly pungent with floral undertones.
Aniseed	Sweet	Sweet licorice aroma with a fruity, warm taste.
Basil	Strong	Deep, rich taste with a touch of mint flavor.
Bay leaf	Pungent	Bitter, spicy, strong flavor; a bit piney.
Caraway seed	Pungent	Sharp aroma, biting, warm, sweet flavor.
Cardamom	Pungent	Smoky, brash, and a little funky.
Cayenne	Hot	Pungent; the chemicals responsible for its heat repel grazing animals.
Celery seed	Pungent	Haylike, grassy, slightly bitter.
Chervil	Mild	Sweet, hints of anise with undertones of parsley and pepper.
Chives	Medium	Smallest member of the onion family. Delicate flavor.
Chiles	Mild to medium hot	Sweet, slightly smoky, and fruity flavor.
Cilantro	Amalgamating	Mix of citrus and parsley.

Cinnamon	Sweet	Delicate spicy, sweet flavor.
Cloves	Pungent	Sharp and bitter with a hint of heat.
Coriander	Amalgamating	Warm, nutty, spicy with a hint of orange.
Cumin	Pungent	Spicy, sweet, and somewhat bitter.
Dill	Strong	Fresh, floral flavor.
Fennel seed	Amalgamating	Warm, licorice aroma, slightly sweet.
Fenugreek	Pungent, strong	Nutty and bittersweet, a hint of heat.
Garlic	Pungent	Strong and spicy with a lemon/citrus, woody, earthy flavor. Sweetens with cooking to become delicate and nutty.
Ginger	Pungent	Peppery and warm with lemon undertones.
Horseradish	Hot	Member of mustard family; hot and spicy.
Lemongrass	Strong	Fresh, citrus, floral flavor. Key ingredient in Southeast Asian spice blends.
Mace	Pungent	Similar to nutmeg; mildly nutty, sweet, and warm.
Marjoram	Pungent	A bit minty, a little sharp, with bitter notes.
Mint	Strong	Refreshing and mellow with lemon undertones.
Mustard	Hot	Family includes black mustard, brown mustard, horseradish, and wasabi. Seeds have a nutty, sweet flavor. Powder is tangy and contributes to the depth of flavor of a dish. It acts as an emulsifier.
Nutmeg	Sweet	Spicy, sweet, slightly bitter with hints of clove.
Oregano	Pungent	Sweet, with a touch of anise.
Paprika	Amalgamating	Peppery sweet with a vibrant color.
Parsley	Mild	Vegetable taste; brings together the flavor of other seasonings.

Peppercorns	Pungent to hot	There is a range of intensity and flavors among the various peppercorns. The taste goes from brash, nose-clearing intensity to sweet sharpness. Fruity, grassy, citrusy, piney, woodsy, smoky are all used to describe the flavor of pepper.
Poppy seeds	Amalgamating	A bit nutty with a light crunch.
Rosemary	Pungent	Cooling, woody, minty.
Saffron	Pungent	Honeylike, earthy taste with a bit of bitterness.
Sage	Pungent	Robust peppery and savory flavor.
Sesame seeds	Amalgamating	Nutty and crunchy.
Smoked sweet paprika	Sweet	Rich, deep flavor with smoky undertones.
Star anise	Amalgamating	Mild licorice flavor.
Summer savory	Pungent	Peppery bite, light herby flavor; a combination of marjoram, mint, and thyme.
Tarragon	Strong	Warm, sweet, anise/minty.
Turmeric	Amalgamating	Mildly sour and bitter; slightly pungent, warm, and musky.
Thyme	Pungent	Piney, smoky flavor.

Fire Up

So far, I have praised spices for what they can do to add powerhouse flavor to what you eat. Now I want to introduce you to spices that can support your weight loss efforts. Spices can reduce your appetite, boost your metabolism, and help your body to burn energy more quickly, which leads to using energy stored in fat, even belly fat. Spices can control blood sugar and regulate insulin, turning your body into a fat-burning machine. When your blood sugar level stays even, you will be more likely to burn fat than to store excess calories as fat. Spices can reduce inflammation and bring your body back into balance. Chronic inflammation has been associated with weight gain and many diseases. Finally, the calming effect of many spices can help to reduce stress-related eating and cravings. You will find "Fire Up" sidebars throughout the book that highlight the spices that can contribute to burning fat and dropping pounds.

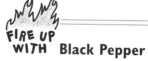

FIRE UP WITH Black Pepper

When see you see what pepper can do to support weight loss, your pepper grinder will become your weapon against fat and extra pounds. Piperine, the chemical compound in black pepper that gives the spice its pungency, can jump-start weight loss. Black pepper:

- Boosts your metabolism, which increases the speed at which your body converts what you eat to energy.
- Continues to increase the rate at which you burn calories hours after eating it.
- Impedes the creation of new fat cells.
- Helps to block fat accumulation.
- Makes you feel fuller.
- Acts as a natural antidepressant to lift your spirits.

Use coarsely ground black pepper to perk up practically everything, even fruits like apples and melons.

Spices That Support Weight Loss

The list that follows provides you with a summary of fourteen spices and how they can contribute to achieving your weight loss goals.

Black Pepper

The substance that gives pepper its flavor is called piperine. It has been shown to help the body burn more calories through the process of thermogenesis. Piperine can also help your body to absorb nutrients more efficiently. Even better, piperine is thought to interfere with the formation of new fat cells. The result: reduced body fat and a smaller waist.

Cardamom

Recent animal studies have shown that cardamom helps to lower blood sugar and regulate insulin. When blood sugar levels are steady, you won't have the same level of hunger as you do when your blood sugar is low.

Cayenne Pepper

If you eat cayenne pepper three times a day, the active compound in the spice increases the rate at which you burn fat. The capsaicin compound in cayenne stimulates your brain to release endorphins, the brain's feel-good chemicals.

Chile Peppers

Capsaicin is also what gives chile peppers their kick. The compound has been shown to increase thermogenesis, reduce belly fat, and suppress appetite. It also boosts the body's ability to burn food as energy. One study shows that men who ate spicy appetizers ate 200 fewer calories at later meals than those who did not.

Cinnamon

Cinnamon stabilizes blood sugar levels and improves insulin sensitivity. A powerful antioxidant and anti-inflammatory, cinnamon is one of the top fat-burning spices. Some studies have shown that cinnamon can reduce the accumulation of belly fat.

Cloves

Cloves can contribute to your weight loss by boosting your metabolism so you burn more calories.

Coriander

Coriander, which is used in many Indian spice mixes, has been shown in animal studies to increase metabolic function and increase weight loss.

Cumin

Though cumin has not been studied by itself, it can improve weight loss when mixed with other herbs and spices. Think of curries and chili.

Garlic

Garlic appears to help your body metabolize carbohydrates and fats more efficiently. It contains phytochemicals that break down fat deposits. Some animal studies have shown that garlic may prevent the body from creating more fat.

Ginger

Ginger is known to reduce appetite and cut cravings. Studies suggest that ginger may accelerate the rate at which the stomach empties. Ginger can boost your metabolism by about 20 percent for three hours.

Mustard

This spice has a thermogenic effect, which causes your body to burn more calories as you digest food. If you want to intensify the effect, try seasoning your food with powdered mustard seed. One study showed that 1 teaspoon of spicy or whole grain mustard increased metabolism by up to 25 percent for several hours after eating. Another study showed that eating ¾ teaspoon of powdered mustard seeds a day burns an extra forty-five calories an hour.

Parsley

Parsley can reduce your levels of blood glucose, as blood sugar is called. Reducing blood sugar levels can help to control your appetite and make the processing of food into energy more efficient.

Peppermint

The smell of peppermint can decrease your appetite.

Turmeric

This spice helps to reduce inflammation, which is one of the root causes of weight gain and obesity. It is also an antioxidant, which protects your body from damaging free radicals that cause an inflammatory response. Animal studies have shown turmeric to prevent the growth of fat tissue.

In the continuing story of my battle with my weight, I zeroed in on spices and herbs to create layers of flavor in the food I cooked. The taste of my food was so satisfying it helped me to conquer my cravings and forget about junk food, well, most of the time. When I saw how my approach to food had positive results for others, including Steve Harvey, I realized I had found a way to eat that hit the bliss point by indulging the taste buds with wholesome food prepared in a healthy way.

My aim in this chapter was to familiarize you with the herbs and spices that saved my life. I have described their characteristics, so that the spice rack is not a mystery to you and you have a richer understanding of what the contents of those jars bring to food. This chapter has laid the foundation for your becoming an architect of flavor. I have also targeted a number of "fire up" spices that can support your weight loss with their medicinal effects.

In the next chapter, I examine compulsive overeating and food addiction and how junk food hijacks your brain to create food cravings. I introduce you to nine diet personalities that reflect what you crave most and how you tend to eat. I have to confess right now that I can identify with all nine personalities!

3

JUST CAN'T STOP EATING

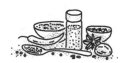

When I was feeling bad about myself for being overweight, I was bombarded by images of thin, sexy people living their flawless lives in magazines, on TV, in music videos, and in the movies, which made me feel worse. I hated myself for not looking and living the way they did. Almost everyone I saw seemed to be in better shape than I was. In comparison, I was so bulky and unhappy. I felt so isolated. Now I know I was far from alone. The fact is, there is an epidemic of overweight and obesity in the United States.

An estimated 160 million Americans are either overweight or obese. Let me clarify the difference between the two. If your weight is 10 to 20 percent more than what it should be, you are overweight. When your weight is 20 percent or more above what it should be, the label "obese" applies. There are charts and free calculators available online to give you an idea of the weight range you should be in.

The statistics about how widespread weight problems are in the United States are alarming:

- More than two in three adults are overweight or obese.
- Nearly three out of four men are overweight or obese.
- Nearly three out of five women are overweight or obese.
- More than one in three adults—78 million—have obesity.

- One in three children under the age of twenty are overweight or obese, up from one in five children in 1980.
- More than one in six children under the age twenty have obesity.

I was especially upset to learn from reports of the Centers for Disease Control that non-Hispanic blacks have the highest rates of obesity at 48.1 percent. Hispanics are at 42.5 percent, non-Hispanic whites at 34.5 percent, and non-Hispanic Asians at 11.7 percent. These numbers mean that roughly one out of two African Americans, two out of five Hispanics, one out of three whites, and one out of ten Asians are obese.

I have included these statistics to assure you that millions of people struggle with their weight just as you do. There are twice as many overweight people in this country as there are people of normal weight. Although there may be comfort in numbers, this doesn't mean you should give up. Understanding the patterns of your eating behavior and the physical process that causes you to overeat will help you to take steps to put on the brakes.

FROM COMPULSIVE OVEREATING TO ADDICTION

Everyone eats too much now and then. Think about how stuffed you were after Thanksgiving dinner, yet you found room for another piece of pecan sweet potato pie, made with bourbon, of course. Or maybe you ate an entire pint of rich, salted caramel ice cream right out of the container after a bad day at work or for no reason at all. The issue is how often you overeat. If eating becomes your go-to way of coping, that occasional binge eating can evolve into food addiction.

You might be familiar with some of the feelings and behaviors I described in my own story of full-out food addiction. There is a continuum of behavior in people's relation to food, from normal to addicted, with differences of degree ranging along the spectrum. You might be so worried about gaining weight that you hardly eat anything. You might simply stop eating when you are no longer hungry. If that is the case, you are one of the lucky ones and probably do not have much of a weight problem. You might allow yourself to binge occasionally in response to something upsetting, but eat normally most of the time. Maybe you binge and purge now and then. Or you might have a binge-eating disorder. You eat large amounts of food compulsively and feel guilty afterward. In order to be diagnosed with the disorder, you have to binge at least once a week over a period of at least three months. But not everyone who overeats is a binger. You might skip meals and pick at food all day long when you are feeling upset or lonely. You might make a habit of eating small meals all day rather than having three set meals. Grazing is an easy way to overeat. Or you could be totally out of control as I was. I could never eat enough to feel full.

This is a good time to evaluate the extent of your problems with food. When you read the following list of signs of compulsive eating and addiction, be honest with yourself about your eating habits and how you regard your weight:

- You think about food and/or your weight all the time.
- Your weight fluctuates. You try one diet after another, lose weight, and put it back on.
- Sometimes you want to stop eating and find that you can't. You keep going back for more.
- You hold back when you eat with other people and tend to eat more when you are alone.
- You eat large amounts of food at one time, often more rapidly than normal.
- You eat when you are not hungry.
- You eat to escape your feelings.
- You eat in secret sometimes.
- You have hidden food to make sure you have enough.
- You often feel guilty and ashamed about what and how much you've eaten.
- You are too self-conscious to participate in physical activities such as dancing or sports.
- You believe your life will be better or your real life will begin when you lose the weight.
- You think that food is your only friend.
- You feel hopeless about changing your relationship with food.

If you can relate to some of these points, you may be a compulsive eater, a food addict, or on your way to becoming one. The label does not matter.

What matters is that you recognize the issues and change your eating habits to healthy ones.

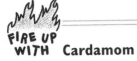

FIRE UP WITH Cardamom

This exotic spice has been used to treat obesity in India for hundreds of years. Cardamom helps your body burn calories faster and boosts fat burning. It aids with digestion as well.

The spice is used in many Indian blends for curry, but its spicy-sweet flavor can be good in baked goods and fruit pies.

Mix a teaspoon of crushed cardamom with green tea for a refreshing weight loss tea.

Sugar, fat, salt, and flour affect your brain in the same way alcohol, nicotine, heroin, and cocaine do. Eating highly processed foods, which contain a large measure of sugar, salt, fat, and flour, can change your brain chemistry and create cravings. Eating too much highly refined food can also override your body's appetite controls and lead you to overeat.

The manufacturers of junk food design their products to be as addicting as possible, just like cigarettes. Processed foods have a hidden power to make you feel hungrier. The more refined or processed food is, the more addictive it can become.

Sugar is especially addictive, and the average American is eating a lot more sugar today than in the past. In fact, the average person's sugar consumption doubled in the United States during the twentieth century. In 1909, individuals consumed 80 pounds of added sugar a year. By 1999, sugar consumption per person was up to 152 pounds a year; 64 pounds of that total comes from high-fructose corn syrup found in processed foods and soda.

Our eating habits have changed. We are eating out more and saving time by eating prepared food. Refined flour, artificial sweeteners, and cereal products began to be heavily marketed in the 1960s. White flour affects blood sugar in the same way sugar does, because flour quickly breaks down to sugar in the body. A slice of white bread has the same effect on the body as five teaspoons of sugar, and two slices equal the sugar in a can of soda.

I Actually Love This Cooking Thing Now

I gave birth to my second child in the beginning of 2015 and found it more difficult to lose the baby weight this time around. I stayed exhausted and now had to manage a full household. The most convenient way to eat was via restaurants, takeout, and drive-thrus.

When I attended Judson's cooking demo at the National Association of Health Services Executives conference in October of 2015, my idea of healthy eating changed forever. I left inspired to kick the habit of eating out five to six days a week and to focus instead on preparing fresh food at home using the right spices to make the food enjoyable. I even got my husband, who had also gained weight, to commit, which was like pulling teeth!

We came up with a routine to shop, cook, and take care of the kids. We started Phase 1 in January 2016. In the first two weeks of applying the Spice Diet, I lost five pounds. To date, I have lost a total of fifteen pounds in a little over two months. I credit a large part of this to omitting the fast food and bringing on the flavor to nourishing dishes. I actually love this cooking thing now! I am dedicated to continuing Phase 1 until I lose another ten pounds and then I am ready to keep it all off this time around.

—*Tanya S.*

The epidemic of rising weight in this country parallels the increased consumption of convenience food, which is highly processed. "Hyperpalatable food" is everywhere, easily accessible, and inexpensive. Frozen dinners, canned soups, and just about anything that comes in a bag or a box are chock-full of sugar, salt, and fat to make them taste better—and let's not forget the preservatives and other chemicals that are added. The Spice Diet calls for you to replace processed food with healthy, natural food, which you make yourself with spices and herbs for flavor instead of sugar, salt, and unhealthy fat. Processed food is so overflavored that you will need to retrain your taste buds and restore your sensitivity to natural flavors. The Spice Diet will help you with that.

The Making of a Food Craving

I don't want to overwhelm you with too much scientific information, but I think it is important for you to understand how you develop cravings. You will see how overeating actually changes your brain. When you eat processed food frequently, you eventually need more food to feel satisfied.

The junk food you eat triggers the reward circuit in your brain, which involves pleasure, memory, and motivation. The human brain registers all pleasures in the same way: A martini, addictive drugs, sex, winning a championship, or a sumptuous feast can all set off the same response. The brain first releases "feel good" chemicals, including serotonin and endorphins, from its pleasure center.

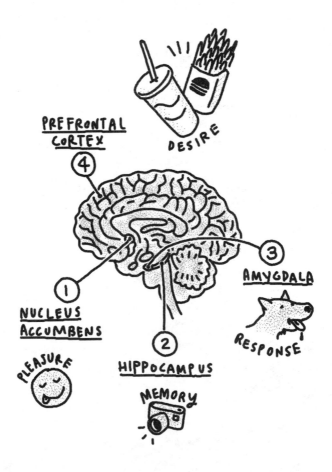

Highly processed food takes a shortcut to the brain's reward center by flooding the nucleus accumbens, a cluster of nerve cells in the middle of the brain that lies underneath the cerebral cortex, with the neurotransmitter dopamine, an endorphin that causes you to experience pleasure. The hippocampus lays down memories of this rapid sense of satisfaction, and the amygdala creates a conditioned response to the food. Finally, the prefrontal cortex produces the craving by combining the memory of liking the food to wanting it.

An addictive substance like sugar can cause the reward center to produce two to ten times more dopamine than usual, which makes the experience very pleasurable, very quickly. Many types of processed foods are designed to flood your brain with dopamine.

The dopamine released in response to the treat you just ate interacts with another neurotransmitter, called glutamate, which controls the reward-learning center. The hippocampus creates a memory of this rush of satisfaction. This is an important function of your brain, because the system links activities needed for human survival, such as eating and sex, with pleasure and reward, causing a memory to be formed. It does the same for addictive substances.

Then the amygdala, which is involved with emotions, creates a conditioned response, which connects the emotional memory of feeling good with that treat.

And now cravings originate: Repeated exposure to an addictive substance causes nerve cells in the nucleus accumbens and the prefrontal cortex, the area of the brain involved in planning, to combine liking something with wanting it, driving you to go after it. This process motivates you to take action to seek the source of pleasure. With food cravings, you want to re-create the pleasurable sensation and relate the feeling to eating.

Over time, the experience of that food becomes less pleasurable, because your brain produces a reduced amount of dopamine or the dopamine receptors are not as responsive. When this happens, dopamine has less impact on the reward center. You have to consume more of the food, because your brain has adapted. You build a tolerance to what used to flood your brain with dopamine. The pleasurable impact of the substance is weaker, but the memory of the desired effect and the need to create that feeling continues unaltered. These memories produce a conditioned response—and you experience the intense craving known as addiction.

I have explained the process to you so you can see that willpower does not have a lot to do with succumbing to a craving. By eating junk food repeatedly, you can change the biology of your brain and set a vicious cycle in motion that is difficult to stop. The more processed food you eat, the more you will want.

To cut off your addiction to food that is bad for you, you have to eat fresh, whole food that is seasoned to excite your brain. The recipes and the spice blends I have created for *The Spice Diet* will do just that, because they provide a balance of flavors—sweet, salty, sour, savory, and bitter—that will satisfy all your taste buds.

I am not someone who has never experienced the tumultuous roller coaster of food addiction; I know what a vicious and debilitating cycle it can be. So, as the "architect of flavor," I can assure you that these healthy recipes will ignite explosions in your mouth and brain. When what you cook is flavored and fired up with the right herbs and spices, your pleasure center will be busy when you eat the delectable food you make.

Pick Your Poison

Most of us crave a particular type of food or flavor most often. Would you call yourself a sweet, salty, or spicy person? Do you crave crispy or soft food? When you have an urge to eat something, what is it most likely to be? A box of chocolate truffles? A bag of BBQ chips? Pralines and cream ice cream with hot caramel sauce? A piece of deep-dish pepperoni pizza with extra cheese? Lemon bars or brownies? A juicy double bacon cheeseburger with all the trimmings, a side of chili cheese fries, and a large soda?

We all have food yearnings that possess us when we least expect it or when we are most vulnerable. I can remember sneaking out in the middle of the night to buy some candy bars at the twenty-four-hour convenience store at the gas station, which was not one of my better moments. If you analyze your most common cravings and the way you tend to eat, you can identify your diet personality. I'm reasonably confident that you will relate to at least one of the personalities described below. To keep it completely real, I was a split personality because I could identify with every type described below. My diet personality changes like the weather. The diet types, which I know all too well, are:

The Chocoholic

You dream about chocolate and wake up thinking about it. You'll take it in any form—dark, milk, or white will do fine. Your goal is to sample chocolate from around the globe. Whether a luxury brand or mass produced from the candy aisle in the supermarket, it's still chocolate to you. You never share your chocolate. You make sure you have a small stash in your desk and in the pantry, where you hide it behind the old "hand-me-down" appliances that simply don't work but have a place on the shelf for sentimental reasons. That's the secret place where no one can find it. You never gulp down your chocolate. You prefer to savor it and let it melt in your mouth. It makes you feel so much better when you're sad. You read somewhere that chocolate is good for you.

The Deep-Fried Fanatic, aka the Drive-Thru Junkie

You have an encyclopedic knowledge of the menus at every place that serves food from a window. Everything you eat needs to come with a side of fries. You usually grab a bite when you are on the go. A slice of pizza, crispy chicken tenders, a couple of hot dogs, or a loaded burrito, washed down with a jumbo soda, and you are good to go. You hate to cook because it takes too long and never tastes quite as good as something that comes from a greasy bag.

The Fizzy-Drink Enthusiast

You could go through multiple two-liter bottles of sugary soda a day. You start the day by gulping down a cold can of soda to quench your thirst, followed by a coffee chaser to rev you up. As the day goes on, you wash down your food with super-sized sugary drinks. You rely on the kick you get from the caffeine in colas. Wherever you are, an open can of soda is nearby. The problem is that the more you drink, the thirstier you get. You've convinced yourself that drinking a lot of fluids fills you up. You reason that if drinking a lot of water makes you feel fuller, then bubbly soda should do even better.

When you read about all the added sugar in soda, you switched to diet soda, which has the same kick. Why waste calories on a beverage, right?

You see no reason to put a limit on how much diet soda you drink, because it doesn't have a single calorie. By eliminating all the calories soda used to add to your diet, you feel you have more leeway in what you eat. You are voracious all the time and reach for another can of soda in an attempt to kill your food cravings. You are sure that the pounds will soon melt away.

The Foodie

Nothing but the richest, creamiest, and most decadent foods will do for you. You like buttery or cream sauces on everything. If it does not come with a creamy sauce or laden with mayonnaise, you are not satisfied. You always have a pint of heavy cream in your refrigerator. Mac and cheese, creamy soups, lasagna, buttery grits, crème brûlée, smothered pork chops, cheesy enchiladas, custards, cheesecake, and fettuccine Alfredo are the foods you crave. You love good wine and exotic cocktails. Holidays are your favorite times, because the table groans with so many special dishes and the best of spectacular confections for dessert. Your picture of the perfect day is either cooking a multicourse meal for everyone you care about or eating one cooked for you.

The Grazer

You are afraid you will consume too many calories if you sit down to eat an entire meal. If you do need to have to a real meal, you take a couple of bites and push the food around your plate. You read somewhere that it's healthier to eat many small meals throughout the day. From the time you get up until the time you go to bed, you are nibbling on something. You drink five Diet Cokes a day. You start with fruit for breakfast and are ravenous by the time you get to work. You keep individual bags of trail mix with chocolate chips in your desk. By lunchtime, you have gone through three bags, along with two string cheeses and a yogurt. You never finish a salad or a sandwich. Instead, you save the rest for later. You find yourself dipping into the cookie jar. M&M's are your candy of choice because they are so small; sometimes you have gone through a big bag by the end of the day without realizing how much you were eating. You finish your sandwich with a bag of chips sometime before you leave the office. You chew on some licorice as you drive home. You have cheese and crackers as you open your mail and unwind. At dinnertime, you nuke a low-calorie pasta entrée. You're still hungry so you help yourself to a scoop of tuna salad that was in the fridge with more crackers. You have a small dish of ice cream. You decide to make a big bowl of popcorn, because there is a movie streaming that you want to see. Then you need some hot chocolate with a few small cookies to nibble on as you read before you go to bed. Without having had one nutritious meal, you end up consuming more calories than you had intended.

The Gutbuster

Overeating is a way of life for you. You aren't satisfied until you can't eat another bite. You can't remember when you last had a meal and left the table without feeling bloated and stuffed. You just can't stop eating. You feel as if you need a nap after you eat. Although you had a big dinner, you can't stop snacking as you watch TV at night. You're trying to watch your portions, so you get up for something else every time there is a commercial. You tell yourself at least you're moving. Your blood sugar levels spike and plummet like a roller coaster, setting you up to repeat this cycle over and over again. After your late-night eating, you sleep badly and wake up exhausted.

The Salty Snacker

Your cupboards are full of processed foods in bags, boxes, and cans. You could make a meal of the snacks served in the little bowls at a bar. You love salty nuts, crackers, and pretzels. The newest and coolest flavor of chips always ends up in your shopping cart. You've convinced yourself that sea salt or organic kettle-cooked chips are good for you. You nibble on crunchy things all day, which you eat absentmindedly, usually right out of a very big bag. You rarely crave sweets, because they're not your thing. You wish you could put salt on the rim of everything you drink, margarita-style. You reach for the saltshaker out of habit before tasting the first bite of whatever you are eating. You're so thirsty all the time that you gulp down gallons of sugar-filled juice and soda throughout the day.

The Starch Softie

When you eat out, you could devour the entire contents of the breadbasket before you order. You just can't resist. A biscuit with gravy is your idea of heaven. You could eat pancakes or waffles for breakfast every day—maybe for lunch and dinner, too. Otherwise, a bagel with cream cheese or an English muffin with butter and jelly fill the bill. You love Asian noodle restaurants. A triple-decker sandwich on white toast followed by bread pudding is one of your favorite lunches at the diner. If you had your choice, you would always eat the white food on your plate first. You can't eat a meal without potatoes (preferably mashed or deep-fried), rice, or pasta. Your favorite part of Thanksgiving dinner is the corn dressing or bread stuffing and candied sweet potatoes. If you could, you'd move to Paris so you could have croissants and baguettes every day.

The Sweet Tooth

You couldn't start the day without a pecan Danish and a cup of coffee with three packs of sugar. You are incapable of passing up a candy bowl. You feel a meal is not complete without dessert. Celebrations of any kind mean you deserve another piece of cake. When times get tough, you drown your sorrows in a big bowl of ice cream with a side of cookies. You consider sugar a pick-me-up and just help yourself to more as soon as you crash from your previous sugar high.

Do you identify with any of these types? You might relate to one or more of these descriptions. I've known people, myself included, who bounce back and forth among all eight. It depends on how stressed out they are and their overall emotional state. As I've said, there's something about each of the Diet Personalities that resonates with me, but The Foodie and The Salty Snacker ring most true.

But you don't have to give up the flavors and textures you love. The recipes in *The Spice Diet* are designed to cure your food addictions. In fact, every diet personality and craving responds to my plan. I'm living proof, a total testament that the Spice Diet works.

The Drive-Thru Demonstration

I had an overweight client who had the same drive-thru obsession I used to have. I knew I couldn't just tell her how her daily habit was harming her, but I found a way to show her. It was a lesson I had to learn when I was about to change my life.

The client and I went out for a meal, and she didn't hold back. She ordered a double-thick burger with bacon, cheese, and extra mayonnaise. As she ordered, I sat there thinking that, back in the day, I would have ordered the exact same thing. She completed her order with a large order of fries and a super-sized orange soda. While she ate, I pulled up a calorie counter app on my phone. Her jaw dropped when she saw the numbers. She was halfway through eating a 2,500-calorie meal, which had 4,430 mg of sodium, 93 g of sugar, and 45 mg of saturated fat. The recommended daily calorie intake for an overweight woman is between 1,000 and 1,600 calories a day. My client routinely consumed over 4,000 calories a day. Her reaction was quite similar to my own lightbulb moment—"Well, I'll be damned," followed by, "but it's so freaking good," and ending with the classic, "So now what?"

I was glad I could give her some answers

I will show you how to create a balance of flavors that will satisfy whatever cravings you have by stimulating the reward center in your brain big time. It won't be long until you are addicted to food that is good for you, which will enable you to regain control over your weight. You will learn firsthand the power of integrating spices and ingredients to create healthier dishes—leaving you completely satisfied and no longer craving the old junk.

4

THE PRICE YOU PAY

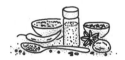

I want to introduce you to Donald "Don" Thompson, the former president and CEO of McDonald's Corporation, and a man I have admired since I was in business school. An innovator with a powerful vision and a creative executive who loves food as much as I do, Don is the current founder of Cleveland Avenue. This multimillion-dollar, state-of-the-art food-and beverage incubator, which helps screen, develop, and fine-tune culinary concepts, is the first of its kind. Don's venture capital firm is a culinary accelerator that brings innovative food, beverage, and restaurant ideas into reality.

Don and I met at a high-profile private event I was catering in Chicago. I always make a point to emerge from the kitchen to meet the guests at these parties. A friend introduced me to Don and his wife, Liz. They immediately told me how much they loved the food I had prepared for the party. They said they had never tasted flavors like those they had experienced that evening. Now, anyone who knows me knows I am very humble when it comes to my cuisine. To have one of the most respected leaders in the business and food world and his wife compliment me on my cooking sent me over the top. I was delighted that they found my cooking exciting.

I was initially a bit nervous to speak to Don, a 6-foot-5-inch thought-leader, whose personal story of how he rose to be one of the most influential people in the world was a testament to his no-nonsense, ardent drive. Me being me, I did not let his position deter me from what could have been my only opportunity to meet him. Don's warmth and enthusiasm for food put me at ease right away. It was an inspiration to meet him. He exuded positive energy and spirit and an overall kindheartedness. I let him know that we were brothers, members of the same fraternity, Alpha Phi Alpha. We exchanged contact information.

I ran into Don again at another party I was catering, which was attended by the Who's Who of the business world in Chicago. He told me about his plans for Cleveland Avenue, which he named after the North Side street where he grew up. He invited me to take a look at the future home of his new business. We met at the 33,000-square-foot building at 222 North Canal Street, which was undergoing renovation. As we toured the raw space wearing hard hats, he talked to me more about what he wanted to achieve. He was driven by the idea of bringing healthier food options to the market. Our visions could not have been more aligned.

Don is known for grooming and developing many people. His reputation as a mentor was unsurpassed. I was thrilled that he wanted to know more about my culinary philosophy. When he asked me to cater a couple of events for him, I knew it was an audition.

He continued to enjoy and be inspired by my food, because he asked me if I would be interested in taking on the role of Culinary Lead and Head Chef of Cleveland Avenue. When Don Thompson invites you to be part of his vision, you thank God and sprint for the opportunity.

I was to help the firm evaluate the viability of food concepts and whether they should be taken to the next level, along with recipe and menu creation and culinary innovation both in house and for our respective clients. Don also asked me, along with our Lead Operations Chef, to bring his restaurant vision to life. Talk about another dream coming true! Taste 222 opened in May 2017 and lives on the ground floor of the Cleveland Avenue building. During the day, Taste 222 is a café with "grab and go" options, serving unique breakfast and lunch items. At night, Taste 222 transforms into an elegant small-plate experience. Our vision was that the restaurant would offer tastes from different cultures and food experiences, engage in cutting-edge techniques, and feature budding trends. The menu can change at any given time and the spotlight shifts to different cuisines and crafted beverage experiences. Guest chefs—from celebrities to underground innovators—contribute to the dynamic menu.

Working with Don has been one of the most enlightening experiences of my life. Having the opportunity to make my approach to food available on such a big stage is a dream come true. And to all of my Spice Diet followers, as you make your way to Taste 222 in Chicago, you will have the opportunity to indulge in some of my recipes and spice blends right in my kitchen. How awesome is that?

I am a blessed man, because I have been able to blend my true life passion with my professional expertise. Having been the leader of the world's largest restaurant chain, I appreciate innovation, trends, and startups. I am dedicated to being an advocate for new food, beverage, and restaurant concepts.

When I met Chef Judson Allen, his commitment to wholesome food and high flavor had already made him famous in my hometown and had earned him praise around the country. From my first taste of the unique flavors of Chef Judson's cooking, I was convinced he was on to something important. There was no question that I wanted him to be an influential voice at my new company, Cleveland Avenue. He has exceeded my already high expectations.

Chef Judson has a rare understanding of what it takes to make food taste great. With healthy eating as the core of his approach to food, he brings his scientific background to use spices and herbs for great depth of flavor. His brilliance has made him a valued member of my team.

—*Don Thompson, founder/CEO of Cleveland Avenue, LLC,*
former president and CEO of McDonald's Corporation

My mentor is as committed to exciting eating as I am. I want to use my platform to help slow the obesity epidemic, which is taking its toll on the health of so many Americans—children, as well as adults. The rising population of overweight and obese people is creating a health crisis in this country and around the world. In the United States, the estimated annual medical cost of obesity-related illness is $190.2 billion, nearly 21 percent of annual medical spending. Childhood obesity is responsible for $14 billion in direct medical costs. These obesity-related expenses are expected to skyrocket in the next two decades, mostly because the growing numbers of today's obese children, especially teenagers, are likely to become obese adults.

Today, obese adults spend 42 percent more on direct health-care costs than adults who are a healthy weight. Moderately obese people are more than twice as likely to be prescribed prescription medicine to manage medical conditions as those at a healthy weight. As a person's weight rises, so do the number of sick days, medical claims, and health-care costs.

These health statistics reflect a grim reality: being overweight can make you sick. I saw the beginnings of chronic disease in myself while I was in college. It shook me up enough to drive me to cure myself by overcoming my food addictions and eating in a way that supports my health—at least most of the time. There is no reason why you, too, can't prevent or reverse illness by changing what you eat and how much you eat. It's never too late to make a difference.

DON'T LET YOUR WEIGHT PUT YOUR HEALTH AT RISK

Scientific research has shown that being overweight may increase the risk of many serious health problems. More than sixty illnesses have been associated with increased body fat. Developing borderline high blood pressure and high cholesterol was my wake-up call to either change my life or be prepared to suffer the consequences. I was much too young to have to deal with chronic disease. I had too many things I wanted to do ahead of me to let chronic illness slow me down.

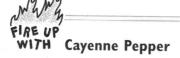

FIRE UP WITH Cayenne Pepper

The active ingredient in cayenne and other peppers is capsaicin, which gives chiles their heat. Capsaicin is a thermogenic chemical, which means it makes your body temperature rise. When your body heats up, it goes into cool-down mode, which burns calories. Initial research has shown that cayenne can:

- Make you feel fuller faster.
- Reduce cravings.
- Suppress appetite.
- Raise metabolic rate for up to three hours after eating it.

If you like spicy foods, you are in luck. Another way to add cayenne to your diet is to mix 1 teaspoon of cayenne with hot water, some fresh lemon juice, and a bit of honey or maple syrup. It's a tasty drink that has been found to reduce appetite while it boosts metabolism.

I am reading you the riot act about the risks of continuing to be over-weight because of the association between being overweight and serious diseases. The best reason to commit to losing weight is to protect or restore your health. Wearing a smaller size is appealing, but it doesn't compare to how good you will feel when you take care of yourself. You don't have to lose much weight to see a positive impact on any conditions you may already have. A modest loss can help to prevent illness from developing. Taking off excess weight can extend your life and allow you to age well by keeping you at optimal health.

Following are some of the most common diseases associated with excess weight:

Type 2 Diabetes

Type 2 diabetes has been linked to overweight. The high blood sugar that is a symptom of diabetes is a major cause of heart disease, kidney disease, stroke, and blindness. Losing just 5 to 7 percent of your body weight combined with moderate exercise can prevent or delay the onset of type 2 diabetes.

High Blood Pressure

Being overweight contributes to high blood pressure, also called hyperten-sion, which may cause heart disease, stroke, and kidney failure. Blood pres-sure is how hard your blood pushes against the walls of your arteries. If your body is large, your heart needs to pump more forcefully to get the blood to all your cells throughout your body. In addition, excess fat can damage your kidneys, which help to regulate blood pressure.

Heart Disease

Heart disease, which is the leading cause of death in the United States, encompasses a number of problems that can affect your heart. Hardening and narrowing of the arteries, or atherosclerosis, can keep the heart from getting the blood it needs. Other problems affect how your heart pumps. If you have heart disease, you could suffer a heart attack, heart failure, angina or chest pain, or abnormal heart rhythm. Being overweight can lead to high blood pressure, high cholesterol, and high blood sugar, all of which may increase the risk of heart disease. Again, the heart has to pump harder to get blood to all the cells in your body if you are bigger than is healthy. The good news is that losing 5 to 10 percent of your weight can lower your chances of developing heart disease. If you weigh 200 pounds, losing only 10 pounds can improve your health. It's a relief to know that dropping just a little weight can improve your health.

Stroke

High blood pressure is a leading cause of stroke, and you already know that being overweight can increase your blood pressure. A stroke occurs when the flow of blood to a part of your brain stops, which causes brain cells to die. There are two types of strokes. An ischemic stroke is caused by a blood clot blocking an artery carrying blood to the brain. When a blood vessel in the brain bursts, depriving the brain of blood, a hemorrhagic stroke occurs. To reduce your chances of stroke, you have to keep your blood pressure at a healthy level.

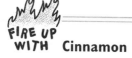

FIRE UP WITH Cinnamon

Cinnamon delivers when it comes to improving your health and losing weight. I consider it a superfood. Using this spice in preparing your food helps in significant ways. For example, cinnamon:

- Speeds up metabolism so that you burn more calories.
- Reduces appetite.
- Alleviates cravings for sweets.
- Helps to burn dangerous belly fat.
- Controls insulin levels and decreases blood sugar, which decreases fat storage.

It is easy to add more cinnamon to your diet. You can mix it into coffee or tea, yogurt, and smoothies, or sprinkle some on fruit.

Metabolic Syndrome

Affecting almost a third of adults in this country, metabolic syndrome has become one of the fastest growing health problems. The syndrome consists of a cluster of factors that raises your risk for heart disease, diabetes, and stroke. You will be diagnosed with metabolic syndrome if you have three of the following conditions:

- Being shaped like an apple with a large waistline. A waist measurement of more than 40 inches for men and more than 35 inches for women is unhealthy.
- High triglyceride level or take medication to treat the condition.
- Low HDL (the good cholesterol) level or take medication to treat the condition.
- High blood pressure (130/85 or higher) or take medication to treat the condition.
- High fasting blood sugar or take medication to treat diabetes.

Since every one of these conditions is associated with excess fat in the body, these health problems tend to occur together, which significantly raises the odds that more serious health issues will develop.

Target Numbers

When you commit to changing your diet, you usually have an ideal weight you want to reach. But the number on the scale isn't the only indicator of your health. There are other measures of health that are equally important, because being overweight can throw off numbers that are critical to your health—like blood pressure, BMI, and more. You should plan to have a complete physical exam before you start the Spice Diet. The test results you receive from your doctor will give you a starting point or baseline against which you can measure your improvement. You should also consult with your doctor about what your ideal weight should be and whether it is safe for you to embark on this diet.

The following chart will give you a reference as to where you want your numbers to be. If you are normal in all categories, good for you! Losing some weight will keep you there. If your numbers are too high, or too low in the case of HDL cholesterol, this chart gives you the numbers to aim for. It often doesn't take losing much weight to improve these numbers.

Health Measures	Target
BMI (Body Mass Index)	18.5 to 24.9
Waist Size	Men: less than 40 inches Women: less than 35 inches
Blood Pressure	120/80 mm Hg or less
LDL (bad cholesterol)	Less than 100 mg/dl
HDL (good cholesterol)	Men: more than 40 mg/dl Women: more than 50 mg/dl
Triglycerides	Less than 150 mg/dl
Blood Sugar (fasting)	Less than 100 mg/dl

Cancer

Science recognizes a connection between being overweight and increasing the risk of cancer of the colon and rectum, endometrium, gallbladder, kidney, and, after menopause, the breasts. The mechanism behind it is not yet known. There is speculation that fat cells may release hormones that affect cell growth and lead to cancer. Eating junk food and processed food filled with chemicals could also affect hormones and cell growth. Eating whole, fresh foods, as I recommend in *The Spice Diet*, may prevent the risk of developing cancer while also helping you lose weight.

Arthritis

Pain and stiffness in the joints of the hands, knees, hips, and lower back can arise from joint injury, age, genetic factors, and being overweight. Extra weight can put more pressure on your joints and cartilage and cause them to wear away. If your body fat is high, your blood may have higher levels of substances that cause inflammation in your joints, which can raise the risk of arthritis. A loss of at least 5 percent of your body weight is thought to decrease the stress on your knees, hips, and lower back, as well as reduce inflammation in the body.

Fatty Liver Disease

This condition is also called nonalcoholic steatohepatitis (NASH). Fat buildup in the liver can lead to liver damage, cirrhosis (scar tissue), or liver failure. Fatty liver disease mostly affects those who are middle-aged, overweight or obese, and diabetic. The cause is not known, but lowering your body weight to a healthy range could take you out of the risk category.

Sleep Apnea

This condition causes you to stop breathing during sleep, which can affect the heart. It has been linked to obesity. A person who is overweight is likely to have more fat stored around the neck, which can compress the airway. As a result, breathing can become loud, difficult, or stop for short periods. When you lose weight, you will have more restful sleep, which also contributes to maintaining a healthy weight.

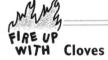

FIRE UP WITH Cloves

Cloves reduce cholesterol levels and regulate blood sugar. Clove water or tea has been used to help people with metabolic syndrome and other obesity-related illness. Some of the benefits of cloves are:

- Increased metabolism.
- Regulation of blood sugar level, which reduces hunger.

Clove tea is a good way to get more of this spice in your diet. Add a teaspoon of cloves to boiling water and let steep. Drinking this tea will help to speed up the weight loss process.

Pregnancy Problems

Before getting pregnant, try to get your weight down to a normal range and be mindful of the weight you gain during pregnancy. Being overweight or obese while pregnant can lead to developing gestational diabetes or high blood sugar during pregnancy; preeclampsia or high blood pressure, which can affect the fetus; the need for a C-section; and a longer post-birth recovery. Babies of overweight or obese mothers are at an increased risk of being born too soon, being stillborn, or having defects of the brain or spinal cord.

If you are overweight at the start of your pregnancy, you are more likely to develop high blood sugar and high blood pressure. Being overweight during pregnancy increases the risk of needing a C-section and complicates the surgery. Gaining too much weight during pregnancy can have long-term effects on you and your baby. You might develop weight problems after the baby's birth. If you are overweight, there is also a risk that the baby might later gain too much weight as a child or as an adult, so you could perpetuate your weight problem to a future generation.

Do not ignore what excess weight can do to your body. You might be fine now, but not losing that weight can stress the systems of your body so they cannot function as they should. Whether you already have health problems or the wear and tear on your body has not surfaced yet, you have the power to reduce your chances of getting sick.

THE HEALTH BENEFITS OF LOSING JUST A LITTLE WEIGHT

You will see improvements in your health well before you are down to your ideal weight. Many complications that could result from being too heavy are improved or prevented with a small reduction in weight. It's encouraging to know that you can start seeing results early in the program.

By losing 5 to 10 percent of your body weight—that's 8 to 16 pounds for a person weighing 160 pounds—you can:

- Significantly decrease unhealthy triglycerides (fat in the blood) by an average of 40 mg/dl.
- Increase good HDL cholesterol by 5 points.

- Losing 10 to 12 pounds can reduce the risk of developing diabetes by 60 percent.

Losing 10 percent or more of your body weight can do wonders for your health. For example, if you weigh 160 pounds and lose 16 or more pounds, you can:

- Lower your risk of cardiovascular disease.
- Reduce the risk of diabetes 80 percent or more.
- Reduce inflammatory substances circulating in the blood, which lowers the risk of coronary artery disease.
- Improve knee and hip function if you have osteoarthritis. For every pound of weight you lose, there is a 4-pound reduction in the load on the knee with each step. An 11-pound loss reduces the risk of knee osteoarthritis by more than 50 percent. Studies have shown that weight loss improves arthritis of the hip.
- Reduce hot flashes caused by menopause.
- Decrease systolic and diastolic blood pressure by an average of 5 mm HG.
- Reduce the amount of abdominal fat by lowering insulin levels and helping to reverse insulin resistance.
- Reduce lower back pain. Adding moderate exercise to your life can reduce the risk of lower back pain by 17 percent.

A New Lease on Life

My female patients always have questions regarding how they can prevent or treat specific issues that affect their bodies. As a physician and nutritional biochemist, I share the Spice Diet with my patients as a supplement to the medical and nutrition education I provide. Diet and weight play an important role in many diseases and ailments that affect women. A healthy lifestyle that includes a change in eating habits can help prevent and aid in the reversal of complicating diseases.

This unique program is safe, approachable, and effective. It helps my ladies not only lose weight, which ignites their self-esteem, but also motivates them to commit to maintaining a healthy lifestyle for the long haul. *The Spice Diet* will give people a new lease on life.

—*Dr. Kenya R. Thomas, MD, MSc*

HEALING HELP

Spices and herbs deliver a lot more than flavor. They can help your body heal. Indigenous populations around the world have known about the functional and medicinal properties of spices for ages. Western science is finally catching up and proving the validity of ancient practices. We now know that certain spices contain potent antioxidants, which protect your body from many serious diseases, including cancer, heart disease, diabetes, arthritis, Alzheimer's, and aging in general. When spices are combined with food, they can boost the natural antioxidants, phytonutrients, and anti-inflammatory power of the food.

A big goal of *The Spice Diet* is to improve your health, and the benefits of eating herbs and spices are an added bonus. When you cook with spices, you are supercharging your food. Powerful spices can reduce inflammation, help to control blood sugar, reduce your risk of cancer and heart disease, and speed up your metabolism. Some spices help to regulate blood sugar by preventing or slowing the production of excess insulin, which stores what you eat in fat. The good news is that when your blood sugar is well controlled, you will be more likely to burn fat rather than store calories as extra weight.

The healing properties of spices are being confirmed by scientists every day. Following is a list of the effects spices can have on your health and the spices that contribute to healing.

Antibacterial: bay leaf, black pepper, cinnamon, garlic, mint
Anti-inflammatory: basil, cardamom, cilantro, ginger, rosemary, turmeric
Antimicrobial: cloves, coriander, oregano, rosemary, sage, thyme
Antioxidant: cinnamon, ginger, paprika, rosemary, turmeric
Cancer Prevention: basil, red pepper flakes, cumin, garlic, ginger, rosemary, turmeric

Chill Out: basil, cinnamon, lemongrass, mustard seeds, nutmeg, poppy seed, sage, saffron, savory

Cholesterol Reduction: caraway, cayenne, cinnamon, coriander, garlic, ginger, turmeric

Control Blood Sugar and Type 2 Diabetes: cinnamon, coriander, cumin, fenugreek, sage

Cure a Headache: cayenne, coriander, mint, oregano, peppermint, sage

Digestive Aid: allspice, aniseed, basil, black pepper, caraway, cardamom, cayenne, cinnamon, coriander, cumin, dill, fennel, ginger, mace, marjoram, mint, nutmeg, oregano, paprika, rosemary, sage, savory, star anise, tarragon, thyme

Ease Muscle Aches: allspice, cayenne, celery seed, mustard seed, nutmeg

Fight the Bloat, Diuretic: caraway, celery seed, chervil, chive, coriander, cumin, horseradish, parsley, tarragon

Laxative: black pepper, caraway, sesame seed

Lower Blood Pressure: garlic, sesame seed

Mood Lifter: allspice, black pepper, cayenne, coriander, mustard seed, rosemary, thyme

Quiet an Upset Stomach: cayenne, ginger, peppermint

Relieve Aches and Pains: celery seed, chiles, cloves, tarragon

Soothe Aching Joints, Arthritis: cayenne, ginger, nutmeg, turmeric

Promote a Strong Heart, Cardiovascular Health: cinnamon, cilantro, red pepper flakes, garlic, mustard seed, turmeric

Strengthen Your Immune System: basil, cinnamon, cumin, garlic, ginger, paprika, saffron, turmeric

Sleep Aid: aniseed, nutmeg, paprika

Harnessing the healing power of spices and herbs, the recipes in *The Spice Diet* address a broad range of health problems, everything from high blood sugar to high cholesterol, inflammation to insomnia.

EVALUATING YOUR WEIGHT ON THE HEALTH SCALE

If you are like me, you have probably consulted charts that told you how much you should weigh based on your height and gender. These measures can estimate your ideal weight and can help you set a goal, but other measures will give you a better idea of your weight in relationship to your health. The three I expand on here are body mass index (BMI), waist circumference, and waist-to-height ratio (WtHR). Calculating these measurements will give you a multidimensional view of your weight that goes beyond the number of pounds measured by your scale.

Body Mass Index (BMI)

Your BMI is a measurement of body fat based on your height and weight, which is a general measure of obesity. You can refer to any number of calculators online to determine your BMI, including:

www.nhlbi.nih.gov/health/educational/lose_wt/BMI/bmicalc.htm

Below are standard BMI charts for females and males for quick reference.

BMI Chart for Women

Height (Feet-Inches)	BMI 19	20	21	22	23	24	25	26	27	28	29	30	31	32	33	34	35	36	37	38	39	40	41	42
	NORMAL						OVERWEIGHT					OBESE										EXTREME OBESITY		
	Weight (Pounds)																							
4'10"	91	96	100	105	110	115	119	124	129	134	138	143	148	153	158	162	167	172	177	181	186	191	196	201
4'11"	94	99	104	109	114	119	124	128	133	138	143	148	153	158	163	168	173	178	183	188	193	198	203	208
5'00"	97	102	107	112	118	123	128	133	138	143	148	153	158	163	168	174	179	184	189	194	199	204	209	215
5'01"	100	106	111	116	122	127	132	137	143	148	153	158	164	169	174	180	185	190	195	201	206	211	217	222
5'02"	104	109	115	120	126	131	136	142	147	153	158	164	169	175	180	186	191	196	202	207	213	218	224	229
5'03"	107	112	118	124	130	135	141	146	152	158	163	169	174	180	186	191	197	203	208	214	220	225	231	237
5'04"	110	116	122	128	134	140	145	151	157	163	169	175	180	186	191	197	204	209	215	221	227	232	238	244
5'05"	114	120	126	132	138	144	150	156	162	168	174	180	186	192	198	204	210	216	222	228	234	240	246	252
5'06"	118	124	130	136	142	148	155	161	167	173	179	186	192	198	204	210	216	223	229	235	241	247	253	260
5'07"	121	127	134	140	146	153	159	166	172	178	185	191	198	204	211	217	223	230	236	242	249	255	261	268
5'08"	125	131	138	144	151	158	164	171	177	184	190	197	204	210	216	223	230	236	243	249	256	262	269	276
5'09"	128	135	142	149	155	162	169	176	182	189	196	203	210	216	223	230	236	243	250	257	263	270	277	284
5'10"	132	139	146	153	160	167	174	181	188	195	202	209	216	222	229	236	243	250	257	264	271	278	285	292
5'11"	136	143	150	157	165	172	179	186	193	200	208	215	222	229	236	243	250	257	265	272	279	286	293	301
6'00"	140	147	154	162	169	177	184	191	199	206	213	221	228	235	242	250	258	265	272	279	287	294	302	309
6'01"	144	151	159	166	174	182	189	197	204	212	219	227	235	242	250	257	265	275	280	288	295	302	310	318
6'02"	148	155	163	171	179	186	194	202	210	218	225	233	241	249	256	264	272	280	287	295	303	311	319	326
6'03"	152	160	168	176	184	192	200	208	216	224	232	240	248	256	264	272	279	287	295	303	311	319	327	335
6'04"	156	164	172	180	189	197	205	213	221	230	238	246	254	263	271	279	287	295	304	312	320	328	336	344

Adapted from: George Bray, Pennington Biomedical Research Center; *Clinical Guidelines on the Identification, Evaluation, and Treatment of Overweight and Obesity in Adults: The Evidence Report*, National Institutes of Health, National Heart, Lung, and Blood Institute, September 1998.

BMI Chart for Men

		NORMAL						OVERWEIGHT					OBESE										EXTREME OBESITY		
BMI	19	20	21	22	23	24	25	26	27	28	29	30	31	32	33	34	35	36	37	38	39	40	41	42
Height (Feet-Inches)	Weight (Pounds)																							
4'10"	91	96	100	105	110	115	119	124	129	134	138	143	148	153	158	162	167	172	177	181	186	191	196	201
4'11"	94	99	104	109	114	119	124	128	133	138	143	148	153	158	163	168	173	178	183	188	193	198	203	208
5'00"	97	102	107	112	118	123	128	133	138	143	148	153	158	163	168	174	179	184	189	194	199	204	209	215
5'01"	100	106	111	116	122	127	132	137	143	148	153	158	164	169	174	180	185	190	195	201	206	211	217	222
5'02"	104	109	115	120	126	131	136	142	147	153	158	164	169	175	180	186	191	196	202	207	213	218	224	229
5'03"	107	112	118	124	130	135	141	146	152	158	163	169	174	180	186	191	197	203	208	214	220	225	231	237
5'04"	110	116	122	128	134	140	145	151	157	163	169	175	180	186	191	197	204	209	215	221	227	232	238	244
5'05"	114	120	126	132	138	144	150	156	162	168	174	180	186	192	198	204	210	216	222	228	234	240	246	252
5'06"	118	124	130	136	142	148	155	161	167	173	179	186	192	198	204	210	216	223	229	235	241	247	253	260
5'07"	121	127	134	140	146	153	159	166	172	178	185	191	198	204	211	217	223	230	236	242	249	255	261	268
5'08"	125	131	138	144	151	158	164	171	177	184	190	197	204	210	216	223	230	236	243	249	256	262	269	276
5'09"	128	135	142	149	155	162	169	176	182	189	196	203	210	216	223	230	236	243	250	257	263	270	277	284
5'10"	132	139	146	153	160	167	174	181	188	195	202	209	216	222	229	236	243	250	257	264	271	278	285	292
5'11"	136	143	150	157	165	172	179	186	193	200	208	215	222	229	236	243	250	257	265	272	279	286	293	301
6'00"	140	147	154	162	169	177	184	191	199	206	213	221	228	235	242	250	258	265	272	279	287	294	302	309
6'01"	144	151	159	166	174	182	189	197	204	212	219	227	235	242	250	257	265	275	280	288	295	302	310	318
6'02"	148	155	163	171	179	186	194	202	210	218	225	233	241	249	256	264	272	280	287	295	303	311	319	326
6'03"	152	160	168	176	184	192	200	208	216	224	232	240	248	256	264	272	279	287	295	303	311	319	327	335
6'04"	156	164	172	180	189	197	205	213	221	230	238	246	254	263	271	279	287	295	304	312	320	328	336	344

Adapted from: George Bray, Pennington Biomedical Research Center; *Clinical Guidelines on the Identification, Evaluation, and Treatment of Overweight and Obesity in Adults: The Evidence Report*, National Institutes of Health, National Heart, Lung, and Blood Institute, September 1998.

As you check your height and your weight, you will find a BMI number that places you on an obesity scale. The weight ranges for BMI are as follows:

Underweight: BMI below 18.5
Normal: BMI between 18.5 and 24.9
Overweight: BMI between 25 and 29.9
Obese Class I (low risk): BMI between 30 and 34.9
Obese Class II (moderate risk) BMI between 35.0 and 39.9
Obese Class III (high risk): BMI over 40

Knowing your BMI can be helpful, but it is a limited tool, because BMI reveals nothing about your body composition and where fat is located. People who have more muscle mass tend to have a higher BMI. Age is another factor that might require a shift in the standard BMI. Older people tend to be healthier if they carry a little more fat on their bodies, but their BMI should not go over 30.

Are You an Apple or a Pear?

Considering your waist measurement along with your BMI will give you a better assessment of your health risks. Where your fat is located on your body affects your health. If most of your fat is around your middle rather than around your hips and thighs, you are an "apple" not a "pear." Men collect more abdominal fat than women. Just think about all those beer bellies.

If you are an apple, you are at higher risk for heart disease, type 2 diabetes, high triglycerides and LDL cholesterol, and high blood pressure. The health risk goes up with your waist size.

Waist Circumference

The Centers for Disease Control and Prevention have stated these guidelines for being at greater risk for developing weight-related health problems:

- Women with a waist that measures more than 35 inches.
- Men with a waist that measures more than 40 inches.

The risk is even greater if your waist measurement is high and your BMI is over 30.

Visceral fat, also known as central fat or abdominal fat, lies beneath your muscles, deep in your abdominal cavity. Visceral fat pads the space between the organs in your abdomen and can wrap around your liver, pancreas, and intestines. Blood from visceral fat flows through the liver and bathes it in products of fat breakdown, which affects the levels of fat in your blood. Having fat around your middle is linked with higher cholesterol levels, higher triglycerides, and insulin resistance that can lead to type 2 diabetes. Belly fat churns out hormones, inflammatory substances, and immune system chemicals that increase the risk of heart disease.

The good news is that belly fat responds well to diet and exercise, but it has to be the *right* diet and exercise. Ab rollers and ab rockers might tighten muscles, but spot exercise will not get at visceral fat. Fighting killer abdominal fat involves eating well and doing moderate exercise along with brief high-intensity exercise. You will find a quick and easy workout in chapter 5 to help you attack this problem fat.

The Ratio of Your Waist to Your Height (WtHR)

BMI correlates with total fat, and waist size correlates with internal fat. The waist-to-height ratio is another way to detect health risk in men and women. The drawback with waist circumference alone is that it does not take height into account. A 32-inch waist on a woman who is 5 feet tall tells a different story from a 32-inch waist on a woman who is 5 foot 9.

Waist-to-Height Ratio

Calculating your waist-to-height ratio is simple: Your waist should be less than half your height. For example, a woman who is 5 feet tall (60 inches) should have a waistline that is less than 30 inches.

When you consider all three measures—BMI, waist circumference, and weight-to-height ratio, you will have more targeted assessment of your weight problem, whether your health is in jeopardy, and to what degree. You should record these measurements along with your starting weight when you begin *The Spice Diet* program. This is described in the Diet Prep chapter (chapter 6). Recalculate these measures as you begin to shed pounds. You will be recording your progress toward radiant health, good spirits, and abundant energy.

5

MIND OVER HABIT

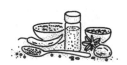

Most Americans equate diet success with how many pounds they lose. Having maintained my weight loss for more than twelve years, I can tell you that the most difficult part of "dieting" is not losing weight, but keeping it off. I have tried countless diets and diet products—from restrictive yet popular no-carb, no-fat, and high-protein diets to moments of despair betting all I had on the ultimate liquid-only diet. I've had the drive to go hard with exercise. The results were inspiring, and the weight seemed to melt away. I was so optimistic that I threw away all of my "big boy" elastic-waist pants and vowed never to wear them again. I was convinced that I had won the struggle.

Within as little as two weeks to a month, I found myself wishing I still had those pants. Once I went off the strict diet, I gradually fell back into my old habits. As my weight crept up, depression and feelings of failure returned. In my mind, I was back in the basement again.

I know what it is like to commit to fad diets, follow the advice of quacks, and believe the broken promises of the self-proclaimed "experts" in the diet business only to end up crushed and disappointed, not to mention heavier than I was when I started. In this chapter, I want to give you my hard-learned tips on how to succeed at breaking food addictions, take control of your eating, and substitute food that is so delicious you won't believe it's good for you. When you do that, your weight will go down as a side effect of eating tasty food that happens to be healthy.

TEN WAYS TO BE THE BOSS OF WHAT YOU EAT

I. Redefine the Word *Diet*

When I felt the hopelessness of my yo-yo dieting, I knew it was time for me to look at the word *diet* in a different way. If you are like me, you have selected a diet to "go on" for a specific amount of time or until you reach your desired weight. When viewed this way, a diet means a punishing period of deprivation and hunger. You have a quick weight loss regimen to follow, which you do for two weeks, a month, or six weeks. When you are enthusiastic about your falling weight, you are able to follow any regimen, no matter how restrictive, for a given period of time.

If you were to calculate the daily calorie count on most quick-weight-loss diets, you would find you are eating 700 to 1,100 calories a day. Of course you are losing weight—you are barely eating enough to sustain yourself. The trouble is that you are not meant to eat that way for long periods of time, and you set yourself up for failure when you do. Every cell in your body reacts to your drastically reduced caloric intake with alarm and kicks into starvation mode. Not only do your cravings intensify, but your body also becomes more efficient with the available calories, which means your metabolism slows down. When you "finish" the diet, your body is primed to fatten up to make up for the perceived period of starvation—the last thing you want.

The first step to diet success is to change the meaning of the D-word. You have been conditioned to see a diet as something you go on to lose weight and then go off once the weight loss has occurred. The weight loss industry is a $60-billion-a-year business encompassing gyms, weight loss programs, and countless diet foods, including diet soda. At any given time, 108 million people in the United States are "on a diet." Most "go on" a diet four or five times a year. How many diets have you tried in one year? As you have probably learned from experience, "going on" a diet that has a beginning and end has done little to solve your weight problems.

As I said earlier, a diet is simply what you eat, a habit. If you want to be healthy and lose weight, you have to look at what you normally consume every day and substitute healthier food options for the junk food. You have to change your diet, the way you eat, for good. That's what I have done. Now, let me be clear: I'm not saying that I don't have a craving for junk food now and then, which I do satisfy occasionally, but I don't go into a food trance anymore.

As you will see, *The Spice Diet* will help you to make fundamental changes in the way you eat. The satisfying and delicious "real" food you will be eating will make junk food pale in comparison. The difference is like a beautiful piece of dry-aged beef grilled to perfection versus a piece of roadkill cooked until it's as hard as a hockey puck. Once you retrain your taste buds, you might find it hard to believe that you ever devoured food designed to make you crave it. Junk food will taste chemical and disgusting to you. I know I was surprised when I was able to drive by a fast-food restaurant without a thought of stopping. Now that was a victory—better yet, it was a miracle!

2. Face Your Truths

When I saw that graduation picture of my obese self at more than 350 pounds and was shocked by the reality of my weight situation, I resolved to change permanently, but there was a major roadblock in my way. I had to face my truths before I could expect to change the key issue that defined my life. I had to meet my demons head on if I was to fight for my life. Doubt and fear crept in. I wondered if I could do it. After all, I had tried to make changes in the past, and nothing I did stuck. I knew I had to get to the source of my issues with food to succeed at change.

As part of my process, I forced myself to dive into my past to get to the root causes of my addiction. This sort of introspection was new to me. I had spent so long denying who I was and what I felt that the process was extremely difficult. It hurt to review the painful experiences and perceptions that had shaped me. I uncovered so much struggle, pain, self-hatred, and rejection that had plagued me when I was young. I grew to understand the family dynamics that had troubled me, without judging or blaming anyone. I saw that all the bad feelings had followed me into adulthood.

I took an introspective nosedive into that jumble of emotions. It was the first time in my life that I broke through the facade I had so carefully constructed to protect myself. I allowed myself to be vulnerable and to go to places I had consciously and unconsciously avoided. I acknowledged that I had been in denial about how overweight I was. I had managed to turn away from that obvious truth. It went the other way, too. My perceptions came from such a hypersensitive, self-critical place that I probably misinterpreted many experiences. I came to realize how wrong I could be about situations. I had kept everything buried deep within myself. I knew I had to let it all go to prevail. I needed a complete cleansing of my mind and spirit in order to reset the way I saw the world and my place in it.

When I finally let the walls down, the darkness inside me erupted, demanding that I acknowledge the negativity and pain I had kept contained for so long. Confronting my inner demons was one of the most difficult things I have ever done, but I finally came to terms with my issues. I was able to forgive myself, as well as those in my life who had hurt me. I stopped playing the blame game, making others responsible for my problems. I knew I had to become accountable for my troubles. I was no longer harboring anger at those I thought had wronged me. On the contrary: I had to ask for forgiveness from those I had wronged as a result of my deep self-loathing. During my soul-searching, I cleared the way for growth and inner light.

If you want the Spice Diet to work for you, you have to face your truths by addressing the issues and emotions that got you to this point. It's easy to focus on the outside—what you see in the mirror, instead of what is happening inside. If you have never gone to this place before, I won't hold back or sugarcoat the reality that it will be one of your most painful experiences. We spend our lives giving advice to others to help them figure out their way. When it comes to engaging in a one-on-one with ourselves, we rarely go beyond the surface. One of the most powerful thoughts we must repeat as often as possible is "I love me." As cliché as I may sound, something as simple as demanding your attention, when you are staring at yourself in the mirror, and repeating it as many times as you need to ensure that you believe the positive affirmations you must speak to yourself. These affirmations provide strength and help you believe in the potential of an action you are trying to manifest. Though this is true, be aware of your internal dialogue and troubled thoughts when you look in a mirror.

Some of my choice words are:

- "I love you, [say your name], beyond measure."
- "I am conscious of my current situation and refuse to let it dictate or mold my future."
- "I am ready for a transformation into a healthier new me."

Binge-eating disorder (BED) is one aspect of associated disorders, which results in a dual diagnosis. Binge eating involves consuming more food than needed past the point of satiety and having uncontrollable urges to eat, even when not hungry. Described this way, BED has similarities to substance use disorders as experienced with alcohol or cocaine, or opiate use disorders, better known as addiction. It does not matter whether psychological or physical dependency factors dominate—the end result is strikingly similar: a loss of control that leads an individual to behave with reckless abandon in order to fulfill the behavior associated with the disorder. Addiction actually produces changes in brain function, which can be seen on images of the brain.

Dual diagnosis is a modern treatment approach that considers a patient on biological, psychological, and social levels. Treatment involves integrating medical, medications, and social work to deal with all aspects of the illness. Parallel treatment is when separate treatment methods are employed at the same time to address different problems. Would you want to wait to treat your high blood pressure until your heart problems were resolved? Of course not. You would want to treat both problems, which are associated. Allowing your blood pressure to spike out of control would place more stress on your heart, which could intensify your health problems.

We have found that integrated treatment is superior to parallel treatment for patients with a dual diagnosis. In the case of BED, strengthening the ability to resist urges to eat impulsively may allow the individual to focus on modifying his behavior, which may be difficult to do without the aid of medication. Consider someone addicted to opioids. Even if that patient is supported by rehabilitation, he will find it difficult to change his behavior while he is struggling with incessant cravings and opioid withdrawal symptoms. Today, medications such as buprenorphine can reduce cravings and allow addicts to use their higher cognitive abilities to change their lives during rehabilitation.

For someone with a propensity for gaining weight, a family history of metabolic syndrome, a sedentary lifestyle, and subclinical depression, the approach would be multifaceted. She may eat as part of her coping mechanism, which only contributes to her weight-related health problems, including diabetes, hypertension, and heart disease. Being overweight sets off a vicious cycle. Fat tissue releases hormones, which hinder weight loss and favor weight gain. The more fat involved, the more your body resists weight loss.

An individual with low self-esteem, who is already self-conscious regarding his weight, may be more likely to spiral down into bad health and psychological despair. From what we have learned, patients with two or more co-occurring conditions, or dual diagnoses, respond more robustly when their conditions are treated in an integrated way rather than with parallel treatment. A psychiatrist may determine whether a patient had a preexisting mental health ailment resulting from psychological and/or social dysfunction. Treatment may then focus on integrating multidisciplinary approaches that are tailored specifically for the patient.

In the case of binge-eating disorders, we have FDA-approved medication that has been found effective in reducing binge, erratic, loss-of-control patterns that result in consuming large quantities of food. Binges are often followed by extreme remorse, shame, depression, and feelings of guilt. These feelings may leave the patient despondent, hopeless, and depressed, but it does not end there. Over time, the depression may cause the patient to self-medicate by eating more as a coping mechanism. This situation of depression with co-occurring binge eating behavior is no different from that of a patient with anxiety and co-occurring alcohol-use disorder. When both conditions are treated simultaneously, we have seen greater success in breaking the addiction and significantly improved health. The treatment may involve antidepressants, mood stabilizers, anxiolytics (relaxing medication), psychotherapy to treat underlying psychiatric conditions, and/or therapy to alleviate food cravings. A multifaceted treatment plan can enable a patient to exercise rational control to stop binge eating. A professor in my addiction psychiatry fellowship liked to quote another faculty member when discussing addiction. Those insightful words are: "Addiction is suicide on a payment plan." Without treating every aspect of addiction and considering the whole person, we allow patients to make those self-destructive payments.

Nathan M. Carter, MD
ABPN board certified, psychiatry
ABPN board certified, addiction psychiatry
ABAM board certified, addiction medicine

Overeating is often a quick fix for pain—emotional or situational. The pain will eventually return, and you will use food to make it go away again. You want to get out of the weight gain spiral. Each of us has a history that led to our current situations—self-hatred, family or relationship issues, fatigue, financial issues, disappointment, and depression all contribute to food addiction.

Food can become a coping mechanism to help you deal with emotions. When you eat, you can be suppressing anxiety, stress, and grief. As you've read, your brain and body become conditioned to crave food for a momentary relief of stressful emotions. Feeling lonely and empty, some eat compulsively to fill that void. If you are unhappy at work, in a bad marriage, single, alone, looking for a soul mate, unable to pay the bills, or caring for an elderly parent, you might turn to snack foods to fill in what's missing, to help you escape the reality of your life rather than trying to improve the situation.

You might be carrying heavy baggage. You could have been abused as a child, cyber-bullied, the object of ridicule at school, afraid of exposing your sexual preference, dateless for the prom, the last to be picked for any team, or criticized by your mother and/or father. You might relive instances when the "perfectly" thin sales clerk dismissed you by saying the jeans you want don't come in your size, or when strangers feel free to insult you as they walk by you on the street. Maybe you are the only one in your family who is overweight, and one aunt always eyes your plate at the family holiday dinner and says loudly that it's no wonder you're fat. Be prepared to experience pain and anger as you look back. I was surprised that the memories I brought up had lost none of their sting.

Pulling back the layers will stir up some tough emotions, but it's absolutely vital to deal with your past before your future can begin. Then you can put your mind to developing healthier coping mechanisms/strategies. You have to forgive and let go—I did.

3. You've Got to Believe

As enthusiastic and persistent as I am, I thought that committing to a change of diet after all my soul-searching would not be too challenging. That wasn't the case. I had been yo-yo dieting for so long that it took me some time to get back on track. As I began to work out my new approach to food, I had the gut feeling that this time would be different, because I was committed in a way I hadn't been before. Maybe it was my health scare or the graduation photo that brought me to my senses. I found I had new depths of resolve.

You have to begin to see yourself as you currently are and visualize your new self. No more personal beat-downs are allowed. To break a habit, you have to see yourself in a positive light. If you have photos of yourself at a more desirable weight, look at them and use them for inspiration. The photos will give you an image of where you want to be in time. You were there once, and now you can head in that direction or begin to get back to where you were. If you don't have a photo of yourself that you like, create one in your mind. Just don't go over the top with supermodel fantasies. I have to remind you that most models were born that way, and most of the photos you see of their perfect bodies have been Photoshopped.

Although you have a tough road ahead of you, there is a big difference between difficult and impossible. Changing your eating habits is challenging but totally doable. You have to devote your energy to change and be ready to fight. When I began my transformation, I vowed to myself that I would not get discouraged if the road got bumpy or if I fell off the wagon.

When you feel you are not seeing results quickly enough or you are struggling with image issues, you have to be your own cheerleader. You have to have confidence and encourage yourself. Be ready to give yourself a pat on the back for every victory—no matter how small.

4. Break Up with Your Current Relationship with Food—It's Not Working

You may at some point have been involved with a love interest or friend who simply was not good for you, or have known someone in that situation. After realizing that your relationship is more hurtful than supportive, you still may have a hard time removing yourself from the drama. As the song goes, "Breaking up is hard to do." You may be used to the situation or afraid of being without the other person. If you don't take action, the problems will only get worse. The same applies to your addiction to food.

Food addiction has to do with how you behave around and think about food. The habits you have formed with food are the real source of your addiction. If you are serious about losing weight, you have to develop a healthy relationship with food. My goal is to guide you to eat properly again; to replace self-destructive habits with self-fulfilling ones.

By now, you have identified your diet personality.

- The Chocoholic
- The Deep-Fried Fanatic
- The Fizzy-Drink Enthusiast
- The Foodie

- The Gutbuster
- The Grazer
- The Salty Snacker
- The Starch Softie
- The Sweet Tooth

Your diet personality reflects your overall cravings and addictions. Of course, it's OK to acknowledge that you are many of these types, as I have. Now it's time to take stock of your strongest food cravings, which you probably know by now. Also, take some time to observe and understand what situations or emotions fire up your food cravings.

It is helpful to write down not only your food cravings but also what triggers them so that you can look at the list to remind yourself to stay vigilant about what causes you to overindulge. Knowing what sets you off can help you to curb the urge to eat.

SUBSTITUTES TO SATISFY YOUR CRAVINGS

Here is a list of some healthy alternatives to the flavors and textures you may crave. Many of these substitute ingredients are found in the Powerhouse Flavor Recipes for Phase 1 and Phase 2.

Chocolate
Natural dark chocolate
    (70% cacao)
Unsweetened cocoa
Cocoa nibs

Sweet
Fruit (especially pineapple,
    berries, melon, dates)

Salty
Lime or lemon zest
Vinegar (this will cause you to
    salivate as salt does)

Starch
Cauliflower (mashed or riced)
Parsnip mash
Sweet potato

Creamy
Avocado
Fruit, veggie, and yogurt
    smoothies
Vegetable purees
Light coconut milk
Quality mustards like Dijon,
    Creole mustard, wine-infused
    mustards

Crispy

Roasted Brussels sprouts,
    broccoli, carrots, kale chips,
    nut crusts

Fizzy Drinks

Club soda or seltzer flavored
    with pureed fruit or natural
    sweetener made from the ste-
    via plant, or pure honey

The Trigger Trio

Food, emotions, and environments can be triggers to overeating. Trigger foods are different from food cravings. A food craving is an intense desire to eat something, provoked by an emotion or situation. A trigger food sets off out-of-control eating regardless of emotion or situation. A food that satisfies your strong cravings can become a trigger food. Trigger foods are usually highly palatable, calorie-dense foods that combine sugar and fat or salt and fat. Cookies, chocolate, potato chips, and ice cream can fall into this category. A trigger can open the door to a tsunami of bad eating choices.

Think about the foods you just can't stop eating. If you open a bag of chips, you have to finish it. You help yourself to slivers of a lemon meringue pie until it is gone. Make a list of your trigger foods. By identifying your trigger foods, you can avoid them. You can keep them out of your home and resist them when you are out.

Trigger emotions are feelings that set off a period of overeating. When feelings such as anxiety, loneliness, or fear compel you to overeat, the behavior is called emotional or stress eating. Chronic stress can cause you to turn to food for relief. When you are stressed out, your body produces high levels of the stress hormone, cortisol. Cortisol triggers cravings for salty, sweet, and fried foods, and there you have it. Stress can cause you to eat more. Unpleasant emotions—shame, sadness, anger, and resentment, for example—can make you turn to food to bury those emotions. You are in a sense numbing yourself with food. Food can fill a void. Boredom, feelings of emptiness, and lack of fulfillment can prompt the urge to eat.

Some of your eating habits likely originated in childhood. Memories of your parents buying you an ice cream sundae after a visit to the doctor or celebrating a good report card with three pieces of fried chicken, fries, and a biscuit can be evoked in adulthood when you use food as a reward. Maybe you remember baking holiday cookies or pound cakes with your mother and eating the cookie dough raw, or learning Grandma's secret to her crowd-pleasing mac and cheese, and of course indulging in tastes as you both create, or Fourth of July family barbecues in the backyard. These nostalgic associations are so positive, they can drive you to eat particular foods to re-create those good feelings.

When trigger emotions drive you to stuff yourself, you must work on better ways of coping with your feelings. Simply understanding the cycle of emotional eating is not enough. You have to take care of your emotional well-being. To do so, you have to find what makes you feel alive and occupied. Rather than turning to food for comfort, do something that engages you and takes your mind off your emotions. Watch stand-up comedy on TV, soak in a bath with scented oils, learn a new language, join a book club, or have a massage. There are so many ways to indulge yourself that don't involve food. Do not hesitate to find psychological help if your emotions are too strong to deal with on your own. There are psychologists and psychiatrists like Dr. Carson who specialize in treating people with weight problems.

FIRE UP WITH Cumin

Cumin can help you break through a weight loss plateau. This is a spice that burns fat. In one study, people who had a teaspoon of cumin stirred into yogurt every day for three months, along with reducing their daily intake of calories, lost more weight and had a decrease in body fat almost three times more than the control group. The researchers speculate that cumin temporarily increases the metabolic rate.

Cumin is versatile. You can add cumin to guacamole, hummus, or eggs. It's great sprinkled over vegetables you are roasting.

Environments can be triggers, too. I vividly remember eating everything in sight during sumptuous holiday meals at my grandparents' house. I never failed to be a "gutbuster" at those celebrations. Maybe you can't resist eating junk food at a sporting event. Those concessions are meant to be tempting. An all-you-can-eat buffet restaurant might qualify you for the eating Olympics. You might not be able to stop yourself from eating the tiny appetizers passed at a wedding reception. I couldn't drive by certain fast-food places without stopping for a big order. When the cashier looked at me with disgust or concern, I pretended all the food I was buying was for the family. Some people can trigger your overeating. A group of friends or a family member may encourage you to overeat.

The first step to resisting triggers is to know what foods, emotions, situations, and people you can associate with overindulging. Be aware of the triggers that shape your eating behavior. Once you recognize the triggers, you can avoid them or learn not to respond by eating.

You're the Boss

You have to believe that you can control what you eat. You can reclaim your brain, so that you do not succumb to addictions, and you can control what you eat. Remember not to label the foods on your list "bad." It is just food.

Your expectations can affect your eating behavior. If you believe you are going to lose control when you are around a trigger food or you cannot resist a craving, you will do exactly as you expect. You have a list of foods that you crave and those that set off a bout of overeating. A mental shift is required to put an end to your compulsive eating behavior. In your mind, you can turn each of your trigger foods into a food that you can choose to eat or not in whatever size portion you decide to have. By reimagining and relabeling the food, the food has no real control over you.

When you feel like eating or crave a particular food, stop and ask yourself if you are hungry. It's easy to focus on what you want to eat and not consider why you want to eat. Take a reading of your emotions and your stress levels. Are you about to use food as a tool for coping? After years of unhealthy eating, you may no longer recognize the cues that signal hunger or fullness. To put yourself back in control, turn your attention to your body.

If you have a craving or are confronting a trigger, breathe through the urge. Just take a few deep breaths. Try to identify the emotion or situation that has automatically made you want to eat. Know that you do not have to give in to the craving or be triggered. The desire to indulge will crop up, peak, and then go away. Wanting to eat your go-to junk food can happen a number of times each day, but be confident that you can resist giving in. If you stop eating junk food cold turkey, it usually takes only twenty-one days to break the habit. Expect to experience withdrawal symptoms for three to five days. As you break your addiction, you may be irritable, tired, and headachy, but those symptoms will pass. When resisting the urge to binge on trigger foods, resist entirely, savor two or three bites and breathe through the urge to continue, or go straight to a healthy substitute. See the "Healthy Substitutes" section on page 118 for a start. I'll also be giving you some healthy, tasty recipes that will be so much more satisfying than a bag of chips.

Keep a written record of the times you did not give in to a craving or managed to eat a trigger food in moderation. When you look at that documentation of your accomplishments, you will gain confidence in your ability to control what and how much you eat.

5. Shift from Mindless to Mindful Eating

Life is so fast-paced today and things change so quickly that we do everything in an accelerated way, including eating. There are multitudes of distractions to shift our attention away from the food we eat. We multitask all day long. We pick up fast food at a drive-thru and eat on the go. We read the paper on our smartphones as we inhale a pastry for breakfast. We eat lunch at our desks and continue to work. We look at our smartphones to check out Facebook as we take big bites from a sandwich and barely chew the food. We have dinner in front of the TV.

If you're like I used to be, you spend more time obsessing about food than actually enjoying what you eat. That's just mindless consumption. When I talk about mindful eating, I mean paying attention to your food at every step of the way—as you buy, prepare, serve, and eat it. I found that reconnecting with the experience of eating helped me to get the junk food out of my life and replace it with much more nourishing choices. Mindful eating had a lot to do with my losing more than half my body weight and locking in the loss. No relapse for me!

When you eat mindfully, eating becomes an intentional act instead of an automatic one. Rather than "grabbing a bite" and wolfing it down, try making your meals a ritual. Here are some tips for eating mindfully that helped me immeasurably:

- Plan your meals and snacks in advance. Eating randomly and on the run is a recipe for disaster.
- Try to eat at a table in your kitchen, dining room, or office. Having "meals" while sitting on the couch or at your desk is out.
- Turn off the TV and silence your phone. Eliminating distractions is essential.
- Recognize when you are really hungry. Learn to make the distinction between emotional and physical hunger. Tune in to your body. When your stomach growls and your energy drops, your body is sending you signals that it is time to eat.
- Don't rush meals. Eat slowly and chew thoroughly. You will release more flavor when you do. You will eat less if you slow down your eating, because it takes your brain twenty minutes to register that you are full. If you gulp down your food, you can do a lot of excess eating before your brain has caught up with your belly.
- Savor what you are eating. Engage all your senses when you eat. Appreciate the color, texture, and aroma of the food on your plate. Pay attention to flavor. Focus on how the food makes you feel. Really appreciate your meal. My recipes in *The Spice Diet* have layers of flavor that are a treat for your taste buds. When you prepare your own food, working with the ingredients as you cook your meals can add to your pleasure and enjoyment of the aromas and textures of your food.
- Stop eating when you are full. You will feel full sooner if you slow it down. There is no need to clean your plate. Small portions can help you eat only what will make you feel satisfied, but not overloaded. I will guide you on portion control in chapter 5.
- Be mindful of how the food you have eaten affects your mood and energy throughout the day.

When you make mealtime a calm oasis and pleasure point in a busy day, you will find yourself eating less and enjoying it more. Those are goals worth aiming for.

6. Don't Set Yourself Up to Fail

When you are setting goals for yourself, refrain from being too ambitious, because you run the risk of quitting if you don't achieve a difficult milestone. Don't be obsessed with results. You don't want to set yourself up for failure. Although we all want instant gratification, patience is important. It has probably taken years for you to gain the weight you are trying to lose. Do not fall into the fad-diet, quick-weight-loss mind-set. Your goal should be to lose one to two pounds a week. At that rate, you would lose roughly 52 to 104 pounds in a year. As the saying goes, slow and steady wins the race. Imagine yourself a year from now!

You have to do a reality check about your expectations. You should have a weight range as your goal, instead of a number etched in stone. Rather than aiming for your ideal weight and having the total number of pounds you want to lose in mind, break the desired total loss down into smaller increments—say, five pounds at a time. That way you will have many successes along the way that will make you feel good about yourself.

To begin, you might want to focus on small, attainable changes that you can control to improve your lifestyle. Learn to create little, positive habits. They add up. It could be increasing your daily number of servings of fruit and vegetables, getting eight hours of good sleep a night, taking a walk for fifteen minutes after dinner, or substituting a salad for fries. When you are successful at making healthy changes in your life, you will feel in control and confident about your ability to form new habits.

If you are consistent, you will hit the weight that is right for you, and you will do it one step at a time.

Backsliding Does Not Have to Be Forever

In my mind, I was obviously set to go when I started my transition to healthy eating. I had been shocked when my doctor called me to report that my tests showed that I had become borderline diabetic. He said the best way to keep my condition from progressing was to lose weight and to eat in a healthy way. I was relieved to hear that I had a shot at reversing the condition before the disease became full blown. I was worried about whether I could change my entire attitude about "eating healthy," which would require dramatically changing my way of life. Honestly, I felt I was experiencing déjà vu, as if I had been in this place in my life before, and I always ended up right back where I started: overweight.

A friend told me about Chef Judson's story and the Spice Diet. Most important, he sounded like someone who understood my struggle. In fact, Judson had experienced the struggle himself. The program seemed like the answer I was looking for.

I got off to a good start, because I was so motivated. I enjoyed planning and cooking my meals. What excited me most was that I had so much variety with the flavors and spices. What I was making wasn't your typical diet food. My weight started dropping, and I was on top of the world. My clothing was becoming baggy. I was delighted to treat myself to some smaller-sized clothes. Then the company I worked for announced it was reorganizing. The CEO was let go and consultants were running the place. No one knew who would stay or who would go.

I ended up working later and later. I couldn't carve out time to exercise. I'd order in the nights I worked late and eat at my desk for lunch. Salads just didn't do it for me. I needed "comfort" food because of the stress. It was burgers, fries, and shakes, fried chicken dinners, deli sandwiches dripping with Russian dressing and mayonnaise, bags of BBQ chips, and all types of pasta in cream sauces with my signature diet soda. I guess I had to save a few calories somewhere. I kept candy in my desk, which I nibbled at all day. I only got up for meetings or to raid the "cookie basket" in the office kitchen. I'd stop at a fast-food drive-thru on the way home. How could I be so weak-willed?

In no time my weight started to inch up. Speaking of inches, my new slacks were getting hard to button. I literally hated myself for losing control. I winced when I overheard one of my colleagues say, "Patty is packing it on again. Guess she can't take the heat." I was convinced that everyone saw my weight gain as a symptom of my anxiety. I was sending all the wrong messages. The more upset I got, the more I ate.

I couldn't believe I was doing this again. I thought my yo-yo days were over. How could I lose sight of the fact that my health was more important than my job? The way I was eating wasn't doing anything to help me. I knew I had to stop being down on myself and do something. I had to take care of myself.

My compulsive eating was doing me in. I understood that relapses would happen, but I didn't have to spiral out of control. I knew the signs. I could rein in those cravings as soon as I started to backslide. I now had a way to overcome my food addictions. I could substitute healthy Spice Diet food for the junk I was eating. No sacrifice there!

I pulled myself together and followed Phase I of the Spice Diet again.

—*Patty K.*

7. Be Easy on Yourself

No one is perfect. There will be times when life hands you lemons. You'll feel exhausted, discouraged, and defeated through no fault of your own. External stresses, along with your body's resistance to dropping more pounds may stall your weight loss, even if you don't revert to your old habits. Stick with it. You can break through plateaus.

Don't be negative and beat yourself up. Your chattering inner voice can yell at you and criticize you relentlessly. A good way to stop negative self-talk is to talk to yourself as you would to a friend. I know I judge myself with very tough standards. I set the bar high, but I rarely hold my friends and family accountable to the same standard. You have to learn to treat yourself with compassion and kindness. You are healing yourself in body, mind, and spirit.

Be gentle with yourself. If you fall off the horse, get right back on. Understand that going astray is normal. When you find yourself in this situation, remember all the effort you have put into the program so far and how much you want to succeed. If you can't resist a craving for sweets, fries, or bread every now and then, it's OK to have a taste. Allow yourself two or three bites of what you crave. Savor each bite. You don't have to devour it all. A few bites can satisfy the craving. If you go off course, look forward, not back. Remember that every meal is a chance to start over.

Rethink rewards and celebrations, which don't always have to involve food. Food as a reward is a habit you are trying to break. For the new you, a treat could be an adventure that promotes physical activity—window shopping at a mall or on Main Street as you think about the new clothes you will have to buy as you get smaller; picking berries, apples, or peaches at a local farm; taking a yoga or water aerobics class—you get the idea. Be generous with yourself and give yourself a pat on the back when you reach every milestone.

8. Be Positive

To break old habits, you have to see yourself in a positive light. If getting on a scale upsets you and makes you doubt you can do what you have set out to do, don't weigh yourself. A negative mind-set undercuts your efforts and almost always leads to failure.

These new behaviors and attitudes will improve your health, extend your life, prevent illness, and allow you to enjoy everyday activities. You are aiming for so much more than dropping pounds. If you focus on those important, life-improving outcomes when you are discouraged, you will be motivated to keep at it.

Stay away from friends and family who enable your food addiction. Some will intentionally try to sabotage your efforts. They might be jealous of the progress you are making and fear that you will leave them behind as you change. Don't let their words and actions get to you. Just smile and refuse their tempting offers of food or respond to their barbed comments with a smile and an upbeat remark.

I remember an acquaintance coming up to me and saying, "Don't lose too much weight. You don't want to look gaunt."

I laughed and replied, "I've got a long way to go to be gaunt. Thanks for believing I can keep it up."

By spinning the negative comment into a compliment, I stayed upbeat and managed to dodge bad feelings.

Instead of being brought down by negative types, count on positive people who will contribute to the emotionally healthy environment you need to beat your bad habits. You want to be with people who believe in your ability to win the battle.

Not Everyone Will Be Thrilled by Your Weight Loss

I had been successful at eating well and was looking good. I expected everyone to be excited for me. Boy, was I wrong! Some people were more interested in enticing me to go off course than in supporting me. When I went out to dinner with the guys, they pushed me to drink some IPO beer with the wings we had ordered. They just wouldn't take no for an answer. One friend poured a tall glass and pushed it in front of me. When I said, "No, thanks," he got belligerent. He asked if I thought I was better than everyone else. He said I was more fun when I was fat. I just laughed it off and didn't touch the beer. Of course, I would have loved to have a cold one.

Another time, at a birthday party, my family made all my old favorite dishes, including my wife's flourless chocolate cake with both ice cream and whipped cream. This banquet was a disaster waiting to happen. I served myself a small taste of everything. Restraining myself was not easy.

My cousin took a look at my plate and said, "Here, let me give you more. You're going to starve if that's all you're eating. We worked hard to make your favorites." She proceeded to heap more food on my plate.

I didn't even bother to protest. Resisting was a no-win situation. A piece of my wife's cake was what I had planned as my birthday splurge. I had been thinking about it for a week!

I tasted everything on my plate—it was all delicious, but I was not going to stuff my face. My cousin noticed as I moved food around to make it look as if I'd eaten more. She said, "What's the matter? Don't you like the food? Eat up!"

I raved about the meal and said I couldn't eat another bite. She kept pushing me, insisting I should eat everything I wanted on my birthday. This was not a loving gesture. She was clearly envious about the weight I'd lost and wanted to break me down. I was embarrassed. Finally, my mother told her to cut it out, that I'd eat what I wanted to eat. Nothing else would have stopped her. I realized that it came with the territory when you made big changes in your life.

—*Rob M.*

When you notice negative thoughts arising in your mind, acknowledge the thoughts without judgment, and tell them to stop. Think, "There's a negative thought," and let it pass on by without reacting to it. Don't let thoughts that bring you down take over. Think about what you have accomplished so far and what you will achieve in the future. Imagine yourself as you want to be. Good thoughts will drive the bad ones out.

9. Get Support

You don't have to go it alone. Having friends or family members who support your healthy eating and exercise goals is important for long-term weight loss success. They can provide a shoulder to lean on when you are discouraged, or they can be a cheering squad when you reach a milestone. They can give you practical support—for example, watching your kids while you exercise. Having a team behind you who understand what you are trying to achieve can be a big help. You should try to talk with two people from your support group every day on the phone, by e-mail, via text, or in person. These conversations will keep you focused as well as let you vent.

Finding a weight loss buddy can make the process easier. If you enlist a partner, a friend, or a group of friends who also want to slim down to join you in your efforts to lose weight, you will be in it together. Having a companion or group can take the loneliness out of your weight loss journey. You can give each other tips, ideas for healthy snacks, and your favorite recipes. It's great to have someone who will exercise with you. When you have a date to exercise, it's hard to skip it and let someone else down.

Someone who is experiencing what you are can be a great sounding board as you commiserate and share the ups and downs of your attempts to eat well or your anger at people's insensitive remarks. You can remind each other that no matter how much you lose or gain each week, your personality, character, and intelligence remain the same. With this sort of support, you are likely to lose more weight and not gain it back. There is strength in numbers.

There are now many online sites with a community of people working to achieve the same goals you are. If you are self-conscious, the anonymity of joining an online support group can be a blessing. These sites can provide you with a lot of tips and support, including recipes, message boards, and chats, from people who have the same goals as you.

These are a few popular sites:

www.thespicediet.com
3 Fat Chicks on a Diet Weight Loss Community, www.3fatchicks.com
Weight Loss Buddy, www.weightlossbuddy.com
Support Groups, https://obesity.supportgroups.com

Daily Strength Obesity Support Group, www.dailystrength.or/group/
obesity

If you search online for "weight loss support," you will find many other
sites to check out.

As mentioned previously, you might find it extremely difficult to confront
past hurts. It can be a dark experience. If the emotions and memories you
uncover are disturbing, do not hesitate to turn to a professional for help.
There are psychologists and psychiatrists who specialize in treating people
trying to break through emotional obstacles to losing weight. Seeing a professional in the field can help smooth the way for you to set yourself free
from emotions and attitudes that are holding you back. My advice for anyone trying to lose weight is to get all the help you can from family, friends,
support groups, and health-care providers who are trained in obesity and
weight loss.

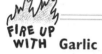

FIRE UP WITH Garlic

Although garlic has many health benefits, including cancer prevention, it can
also contribute to weight loss. Here's how:

- Stimulates leptin, the satiety hormone, which reduces binge eating and
  cravings.
- Boosts metabolism.
- Acts as a diuretic to reduce bloat.

Garlic is so flavorful, you probably already use it liberally in the food you
cook. If you don't, it's time to start benefitting from garlic's "anti-obesity
effect."

10. Make a Vision Board

I'm sure in the past you have dutifully kept a food/diet log at the beginning
of a diet and stopped recording your meals, moods, and cravings at some
point, never to open that log again. It can get tedious and predictable. I think

creating a vision board is a much more effective way to motivate yourself. A vision board is a concrete visualization of your goals. To make a vision board, you select and display images that represent what you want to achieve or how you want to feel in your life. Vision boards have power because they clarify what you want. By creating a colorful montage of your goals, you are reminded of what you want to achieve in a way that focuses your attention. The thinking behind the vision board is that what you focus on expands to become a reality.

To make a vision board, you'll need a big piece of poster board, a cork-board, a bulletin board, or a magnetic dry-erase board. You should find a place for your vision board where you will see it often—for example, near your desk or in the kitchen near the refrigerator. There are also many free apps and vision board software programs that enable you to construct your vision board on your computer, phone, or other electronic devices. The upside of doing it electronically is that you can take your digital vision board with you wherever you go.

Your vision board for the Spice Diet could contain:

- A picture of yourself now.
- Pictures of yourself from the past before you gained weight or were closer to a healthy weight.
- Pictures of slim people enjoying life for inspiration.
- A cravings and trigger-foods list.
- Pictures of beautiful, healthy foods.
- Anything that inspires and motivates you—pictures of your grand-kids; images of people doing activities you might enjoy, like surfing, biking, playing tennis, hiking; great vacation photos; or fashion shots of clothes you'd like to wear.
- Weight loss affirmations—you can find colorfully designed inspira-tional sayings online to print out.
- Symbols that celebrate achieving mini goals—remember gold stars?

Your vision board should be dynamic, so keep some empty space for add-ing more items. You might see a headline that speaks to you, receive a greet-ing card, keep ticket stubs to a sports or cultural event, or pick a flower you want to mount on the board. Your vision board is there to give you positive energy and to be a reminder of where you want to be.

Take some time to create a mind-set that will give you confidence in your ability to take control of your eating before beginning Phase 1 of the Spice Diet. By dealing with the history, emotions, and attitudes that drive you to overeat, you will have a clear picture of what you need to change.

6

DIET PREP

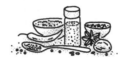

A day in my life as Mr. Harvey's personal chef began at 4:00 a.m. in my home office. I planned the daily menu and curated the freshest, highest-quality ingredients. I sourced the best spices, herbs, produce, and local products during farmers' market season. During the off season, I worked with markets, co-ops, and grocers to get the ingredients we needed. That done, I called my sous chef to go over the details of the day to come. Then I was off to NBC Studios where *The Steve Harvey Show* is taped.

Food prep on site began around 5:00 a.m. We cleaned our produce, broke down our meats and seafood, and started fresh stocks and beans for the day. Because Steve Harvey spends a large part of his day at the studio taping his syndicated radio show and filming multiple talk show episodes, his dressing room/office includes a full kitchen, which he had designed for me so that I could build his flavors there.

Just as prep is a key part of any chef's job, you have to prepare yourself and get organized to achieve the best results from the Spice Diet. This chapter is designed to give you the information and a plan to make Phase 1 of the diet and your transition to a healthier lifestyle smooth sailing.

FIRST THINGS FIRST

Before you start any diet, you should consult with your doctor. If you have a chronic illness or take medications for a medical condition, it is even more important for you to discuss the Spice Diet with a health-care professional to confirm that the diet is appropriate for you. Identify your allergies and other food restrictions in advance. You will find a good selection of healthy food in the powerhouse recipes for Phase 1 and Phase 2 regardless of your restrictions.

It's a good idea to take note of your basic health information, such as weight, height, waist circumference, blood pressure, blood sugar, and cholesterol. Calculate your BMI and waist-to-height ratio. You should record all these numbers on your phone, laptop, tablet, or computer or, if you don't want to go the electronic route, use a notebook. You might want to post them on your vision board. These numbers represent your starting point, your baseline. As you lose weight, you will be able to observe all the improvements you are making in your health. While you are at it, take a photo of yourself as you are now for your vision board or the refrigerator door. The less flattering the photo is, the more motivating it will be. When cravings arrive, you can look at that photo and say to yourself, "No way am I going to eat that junk. I want to change the way I look and feel!"

Going for the WOW Factor

My mom was an amazing cook and prepared meals that I loved, especially her potatoes au gratin. Her chicken casserole was addictive. Having said that, I was living on a mostly carbohydrate diet. My weight escalated to 185 pounds. At 5 feet 1 inch tall, I was obese. I peaked at 225 pounds. Struggling with high blood pressure, prediabetes, and high cholesterol, I didn't have a choice.

I began preparing my own meals, but my cooking left a lot to be desired. When I first heard about the Spice Diet, I dismissed Judson's ideas for getting me in shape, but one day I gave in and committed to give it a try. I saw immediate change as I began to spice up my meals. My food now has that WOW factor. I look forward to cooking these days, and everyone enjoys the amazing flavors of Judson's recipes.

I started losing weight and that motivated me to work out four or five days a week. The good news is that I have lost over forty pounds. I am finally at a comfortable weight of 183 pounds, and I'm not done yet. I will continue to follow this plan until I lose thirty more pounds. When I accomplish a seventy-pound weight loss, I am committed to keeping that weight off. What's great is that I believe I can do it.

—Judy A.

WATCH TELEVISION LESS AND MOVE MORE

Before focusing on what you will be eating, you have to stand up and start moving. Watching television for hours at a time is one of the major enablers when it comes to emotional eating and cravings. Although those food and beverage commercials can break down anyone's resistance, there are even more profound consequences for being a couch potato.

Being sedentary is bad for your health. Sitting for long periods of time has consequences, which scientists refer to as the "sitting disease." Physical inactivity has been linked to metabolic disease, obesity, and diabetes. If you spend your evenings in front of a television and remain inactive for long periods of time, you increase your risk of death from cardiovascular disease and cancer. The *New York Times* reported on an alarming Australian study that found that every hour of television watched after the age of twenty-five reduced the viewer's life expectancy by 21.8 minutes. To put that number in perspective, smoking a cigarette reduces life expectancy by eleven minutes. Other media reported on this study under the headline "Sitting Is More Dangerous to Your Health than Smoking."

Think of how much of the day you spend sitting or lying down. You might spend the majority of your day sitting at a desk, at a conference room table, in restaurants, in your car, on buses and trains as you commute, and then you sit in front of the television or computer when you get home. All the labor-saving devices that are a part of your life can keep you sedentary. You can shop with a click of the mouse, change channels, open the garage door, answer the phone right next to you without having to get out of your chair or exert yourself.

American adults spend 55 to 70 percent of their time sitting or lying on a couch, which would be 7.7 to 15 hours a day. If you add 7 hours for sleep, you could be sedentary for 22 hours a day. It is essential that you move more if you want to be healthy.

When you sit, your muscles, especially the powerful muscles in your legs and buttocks, do not contract. When the electrical activity in your muscles drops, they require less fuel, and blood sugar levels rise, which can contribute to diabetes and result in excess blood sugar being stored as fat. When you are sedentary, the rate at which you burn calories plummets to 1 calorie per minute, a third of what your body would burn if you got up and walked. You do not have to spend two hours a day working out at the gym. It turns out that simply standing more is good for your overall health. When you stand, you burn more calories. Depending on your size, standing may help you burn an additional twenty to fifty calories an hour.

If you are completely sedentary, you might begin by standing more during the day. Make it a habit to get up every twenty minutes and walk twenty feet or keep standing for two minutes. That's all you have to do to start. You can set the timer on your phone to remind you. There are anti-sitting apps you can download on your phone or computer that will let you know it's time to get up. Ultimately, you have to build routine movement into your life. You can gradually add more physical activity.

Ten Ways to Get Moving

You don't have to exhaust yourself for hours at the gym to benefit from moving more. Here are a few simple things you can do:

1. Take a fifteen-minute walk after meals.
2. Play music and dance when you do housework.
3. Stand and pace when you talk on the phone.
4. Get up for water every odd or even hour. As an extra benefit, you'll get hydrated at the same time.
5. Stretch at your desk during the day.
6. If you commute to work by bus, train, or subway, stand for part of the trip or get off a stop early and walk the rest of the way.
7. Park a distance from the entrance of your destination.
8. Hide the remote controls. Change the channel or volume manually.
9. Get up during TV commercials. Do a chore or work out your arms with bands or light weights.
10. Wear a pedometer or an activity tracker. They are great motivators.

You should feel better once you move more, and as you lose weight, it will be easier to move. You don't have to feel lethargic any longer. By burning energy, you will feel energetic. Making movement a habit will help you to tap into reserves of energy you may not know you have, and improve your mood and optimism.

Recreation versus Exercise

Adam Zickerman, the owner of InForm Fitness and author of the *New York Times* bestseller *Power of 10* has designed two high-intensity strength-training programs using resistance bands for *The Spice Diet*. Before you groan at the thought of working out, you should know that each workout takes no more than fifteen minutes, and you only have to do one of the workouts twice a week. No excuses. Anyone can find fifteen minutes twice a week to do these efficient and safe routines.

Before getting into the workouts, I want share the distinction Adam makes between movement and exercise. You need both to raise your fitness level and to reverse the complications of weight gain. Adam considers movement to be recreation, things you do for fun. It could be taking a yoga or Zumba class, riding a bike, playing with children, working in the garden, or taking your dog for a long walk. Recreation restores and refreshes you. As far as I'm concerned, I could use more of that, and you probably can, too.

Exercise in the form of strength or resistance training helps to increase lean muscle mass and reduce body fat. With more muscle, your body will burn calories more efficiently. On a superficial level, you will look better. Muscle takes up less space and looks tighter compared to fat tissue. Take a look at the inspiring bodies on your vision board. If you increase your muscle mass, you will look leaner and toned, which is what you want to achieve. More important than your appearance, when you have a greater percentage of muscle mass, your body will burn more calories at rest. Fat tissue uses very few calories, because it doesn't help your body to move. Building muscle can help you burn as much as 15 percent more calories, which will support weight loss and maintenance.

People who are inactive lose as much as 3 to 5 percent of their muscle mass per decade after age thirty. After the age of forty-five, muscle mass declines at a rate of 1 percent a year. Between the ages of twenty and eighty, you will lose about 40 percent of your muscle mass if you do not exercise to counter the decline. That's why the elderly often appear frail. The good news is that older adults who perform adequate resistance training can increase their strength as much as threefold within two to three months. It's encouraging to know that you can fight muscle loss at any time. Stay strong, and the quality of your life will be so much better.

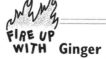

FIRE UP WITH Ginger

This pungent spice is a powerhouse when it comes to weight loss. Two compounds found in ginger, gingerols and capsaicin, are thermogenic. They raise your body temperature. When your body has to work hard to lower your temperature, you burn more calories. Ginger can:

- Increase your metabolism by about 20 percent for three hours.
- Act as a natural appetite suppressant.
- Reduce belly fat by lowering cortisol levels.
- Serve as a mild laxative.

Ginger adds great flavor to soups, marinades, and salad dressings.

Turn Up the Intensity

Exercise creates change in your body and your mind, but there is a new take on how to get the best results from exercise. The latest thinking is that high intensity is the way to go. Adam Zickerman of InForm Fitness is a pioneer in the high-intensity, super-slow movement. His exercise slows the pace of weight training and focuses on fatiguing every muscle to the point of muscle failure. The workouts he has designed for *The Spice Diet* will give you the power to reshape your body efficiently and safely, regardless of your physical condition or age. As Adam has seen repeatedly in the progress of his clients, you can expect to have better results from his fifteen-minute, high-intensity workouts than you would with more time-consuming fitness routines.

Adam has found that the best way to increase muscle mass is to work with light to moderate resistance—or weight—in a very controlled way. When you do an exercise, count for ten seconds as you do the movement and for ten seconds as you return to the starting position. At this slow rate, one complete rep would take twenty seconds. Keep the tension of the movement in the muscle, not the joint. Once you have completed the movement, do it again without resting. Keep going until you cannot move the muscles you are working another inch. As you try to repeat the move, your muscles will burn, and you will shake. At that point, you are in muscle failure.

If you want to see results, you have to work your muscles to the point of failure, meaning you have no more force to give no matter how much you push. Adam calls it "hitting the wall." You are fighting resistance, unable to move another inch. Once you reach muscle failure, keep going, keep pushing. Although you may not be able to make the band move, continue to try for a slow count of ten. That final ten seconds of straining after muscle failure is when the payoff happens. When you complete a fifteen-minute, full-body, high-intensity workout, you have earned time off—exercise-free days.

When you push yourself until your muscles are exhausted, they need time to rest and repair. For proper recovery, your muscles need three or four days of rest. That is when your body begins to build muscle. When you exercise with this intensity, microtears develop in your muscles that need to heal. When the repairs are made, muscle tissue is built. If you overdo the workouts and do not allow your muscles time to heal, you will end up breaking down muscle tissue, which is the last thing you want to do.

Adam says that his clients like to do one workout on the weekend and one during the workweek. He recommends doing the exercises on Saturday and Tuesday.

Keep in mind that you have to work hard to benefit from the rest. Most people stop short of the intensity required for results. The key is to keep pushing until you cannot do another rep and then push for another ten seconds. Exerting yourself in this way for thirty minutes a week will make a big difference in building muscle and burning fat.

THE SPICE DIET HIGH-INTENSITY STRENGTH TRAINING

Before you take on any exercise regime, it is a good idea to check with your doctor to be sure you are able to do it.

Adam has designed two full-body programs of six exercises each to work all the muscle groups in your body. One workout is not more difficult than the other one. He included two workouts because he thinks it's good to change things up now and then. When the routine you are doing gets boring, give the other one a try.

Resistance bands are the only equipment you will need. They are light and portable, so you can take them wherever you go. It's a good idea to buy a set of bands that has varying levels of resistance, because as you get stronger you'll progress to a band with higher resistance. You can use bands that are a long flat strip of rubber. A set comes in different lengths with different levels of resistance. These do not usually have handles, so you can wrap the bands around your hands or hold them farther from the ends, shortening them up, for greater control of the resistance level. Another type of resistance equipment is a set of tube resistance bands, which are made from rubber tubes and usually come with handles. Adam recommends getting a set with foam handles, because they cushion your hands and protect them from blisters. The Spice Diet workouts have been designed to use simple bands or tubes with handles.

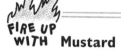

FIRE UP WITH Mustard

The phytochemicals that give mustard its flavor produce impressive weight loss benefits. Eating 1 teaspoon of mustard can boost your metabolism by up to 25 percent for several hours after eating. Animal studies have shown that obese subjects lost abdominal fat when their diet was supplemented with mustard.

There are so many delicious mustards available that you can have great variety. Just stay away from mustards with honey—you do not need extra sugar. Mustard is a must for most salad dressings.

Rather than a set number of repetitions, you will be working your muscles to exhaustion or muscle failure. You will push the initial movement for ten more seconds, or until you cannot move the band, to get the maximum benefit of the exercise.

These workouts are great because you can make them as challenging as you want by choosing the amount of resistance the bands or tubes offer. If you are using graduated bands or tubes, move up to the next level of resistance when it takes you more than fifteen minutes to complete the series. You will know you are getting stronger if it takes you longer to get to muscle failure. Remember: you have to challenge your muscles to get the maximum benefit from the exercises.

Your resistance bands or tubes can be used in hundreds of different exercises. When you are ready to create your own workout, you can find many exercises, arranged by muscle groups, online.

The Spice Diet Workout 1

EXERCISE 1: DEAD LIFT

Target: Posterior chain, upper body, and core

- Hamstrings
- Glutes
- Lats
- Trapezoids
- Erectors
- Scapula stabilizers
- At high resistance: Upper arms at forearms
- At high resistance: Lower, middle, and upper back

The key to doing this exercise correctly is to keep your back straight as you bend from the waist.

1. Stand on the middle of a band or tube and grip each end. Move your feet hip width apart with a slight flex in your knees.
2. Bend forward, hinging from the waist with a straight back. Stick out your butt as you do this. Do not arch your back.
3. With your knees slightly bent, lower your hands toward the floor in front of your toes for a count of 10.

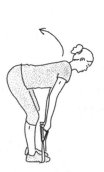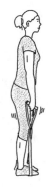

4. With your arms straight, raise your hands as you stand up. Return to upright position to for count of 10.

5. Repeat this exercise to muscle failure. When you can no longer pull the band up, keep trying for a count of ten.

EXERCISE 2: SEATED ROW

Target: Back

- Erector spinae in the lower back
- Middle and lower trapezius in the upper back
- Rhomboids and latissimus dorsi in the middle back
- Teres major in the outer back

For maximum benefit and to avoid injuring your back, be certain to sit up straight with your shoulders squared while doing this exercise.

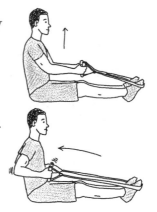

1. Sit on the floor with your legs extended in front of you. Wrap the resistance band or tube securely under your feet. Hold the band at a point that allows you to sit up straight.

2. Pull the band to each side of your torso in a rowing motion with your elbows bent close to your sides until your shoulder blades squeeze together.

3. Pause in this position and then return to start with your back remaining straight.

4. Repeat until muscle failure and you cannot do another one. Then try to pull back for 10 seconds more, even if the band does not budge.

EXERCISE 3: FLY

Target: Chest

- Pectoralis major
- Deltoids

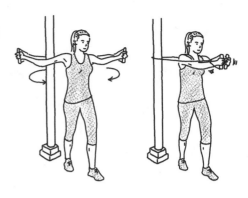

1. Either loop the resistance band or tube around a stable object, such as a pole, anchor it to a door (if your set has anchors), or simply run it behind your back. If you loop the band behind your back, you will probably need to wrap the band around your hand or forearm in order to get enough resistance.

2. Hold the ends of the resistance band or handles in each hand and spread your arms out straight to the side in a T position. Your arms should be just below shoulder height. Be sure not to lock your elbows.

3. Keeping your elbows slightly bent, inhale as you bring both arms forward until your hands meet in front of your chest.

4. Exhale as you return to starting position.

5. Repeat until muscle failure. Then continue trying to move your arms forward in front of you for a count of 10.

EXERCISE 4: LATERAL RAISE

Target: Shoulders

■ Deltoids

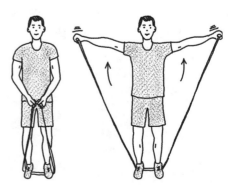

1. Stand on a resistance band or tube while holding each end or handle so that the tension begins at arm's length. Your palms should be facing each other in front of your thighs, knuckles to the floor. Your arms should be fully extended toward the floor with a slight bend in your elbows.

2. Take a deep breath. As you exhale, lift the ends of the band until they are slightly below your

shoulders. You can slightly tilt your wrist as if you were watering plants. Keep your arms extended with your elbows higher than your hands.

3. Lower the handles slowly to the starting position.
4. Repeat the up-and-down movement until muscle failure. Then continue to try to lift your arms for a count of 10.

EXERCISE 5: MONKEY

Target: Oblique abdominals

- Deltoids
- Biceps

1. Stand on a resistance band with your feet shoulder width apart and your hands holding the ends of the band or the handles with your palms facing your thighs.
2. Slightly bend your knees and squat down as if you are going to sit. Your butt drops back slightly as you lower.
3. Bend your torso to the left as you bring up your right elbow.
4. Return to center, then lean to the left again.
5. When you can no longer move the band, continue trying for a count of 10.

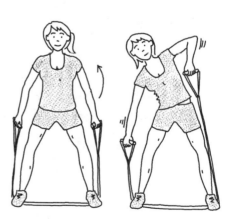

6. Repeat the exercise on the other side. Bend to the right with your left elbow lifted, return to center, then bend to the right.
7. Repeat until you can no longer move the band.

EXERCISE 6: STANDING BICEP CURL

Target: Biceps

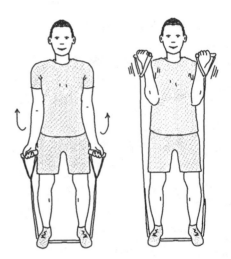

1. Stand on the middle of the band holding the ends of the band or the handles in your hands. With your palms facing forward, keep your hands at your hips.
2. Bend your elbows and slowly raise your hands to your shoulders for a count of 10. Make sure to keep your back straight and your abdominal muscles engaged so you are working your core as well.
3. Lower your arms slowly with control for a count of 10.
4. Repeat the up-and-down movement to muscle failure. Then continue to try to lift your hands for a count of 10.

The Spice Diet Workout 2

EXERCISE 1: LEG PRESS

Target: Quadriceps

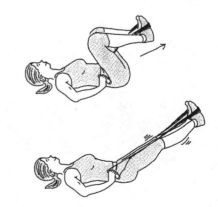

- Gluteus maximus
- Hamstrings

1. Sit on a mat or carpeted area and wrap the band under the arches of your feet.
2. Roll down until your back is flat on the floor.

3. Hold the band or tube by the handles or increase resistance by holding the bands higher with less slack.

4. Bend your knees toward your chest and hold them in tabletop position—your knees are pointing at the ceiling and your shins are parallel to the ceiling.

5. Press through your feet to straighten your legs for a count of 10. Avoid arching your back by pulling your belly button into your spine.

6. While keeping your abs tight, return to the starting position for a count of 10.

7. Repeat the movement until muscle exhaustion. Then try to push your legs out for a count of 10.

EXERCISE 2: KICKBACK

Target: Butt

- Gluteus maximus
- Hamstrings

1. Place the resistance band or tube around the bottom of your right foot and get down into an all-fours/hands-and-knees position.

2. Kick back and up with your right foot as you straighten your leg for a count of 10.

3. Resisting the band, slowly lower your right leg and bring your knee to the floor returning to starting position for a count of 10.

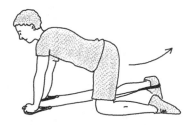

4. Repeat until muscle failure. Then continue trying to push your leg out for a count a 10.

5. Put the resistance band around your left foot and repeat the exercise as you did for your right leg.

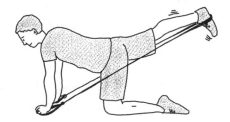

EXERCISE 3: SHRUGS

Target: Upper back

- Trapezius
- Rhomboid major
- Levator scapulae

1. Stand on the middle of the resistance band or tube and hold each end in your hands. Make sure there is no slack in the band. To get the right level of resistance you might have to shorten up the band by gripping farther from the end and wrapping it around your hand.

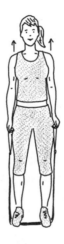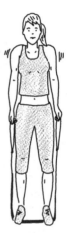

2. Keeping your arms straight, shrug your shoulders up and backward, working against the resistance of the band for a count of 10.

3. Lower your shoulders to the start position for a count of 10. Repeat the movement until muscle failure. Then continue trying to lift your shoulders for a count of 10.

EXERCISE 4: TRICEPS KICKBACK

Target: Triceps, upper back, and rear shoulders

- Triceps
- Trapezius
- Latissimus dorsi
- Rhomboids

1. Stand on the middle of the band or tube, feet shoulder width apart, and hold an end of the band or tube in each hand with your palms facing behind you.

2. Bend over at your waist so that your chest is parallel to the floor, your elbows bent behind you, and your hands up at chest level.

3. Reach your hands behind you and lock your elbows for a count of 10.

4. Return to bent elbows for a count of 10.

5. Repeat this motion until muscle failure. Then continue trying to extend your arms for an additional count of 10.

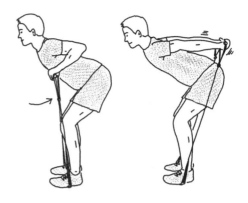

EXERCISE 5: CHEST PRESS

Target: Front of chest and arms

- ▪ Pectoralis major
- ▪ Anterior deltoids
- ▪ Triceps

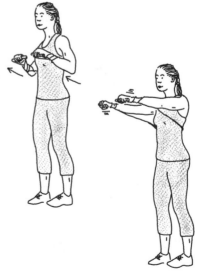

1. You can anchor your band or tube in a door if you have a set with an anchor or wrap it around a weight-bearing pole, such as a metal stair rail. The safest way to do this exercise is to place the band behind your back at chest height and to wrap any excess length around your forearms.

2. With elbows at your sides and your arms parallel to the floor at a 90-degree angle, push straight out for a count of 10. Be sure to keep your shoulders down.

3. Resist the band as you return to a starting position for a count of 10.

4. Repeat the movement until muscle failure and you cannot do any more reps. Then try to push out for a count of 10 even though the band will not move.

EXERCISE 6: LYING STRAIGHT LEG RAISES

Target: Hips and lower abdomen

- ▪ Hip flexors
- ▪ Abs

1. Lie flat on your back on a mat or a rug. Wrap the middle of the band around the soles of both feet. Hold the ends of the resistance band or tube in each hand.

2. Raise your legs to a little less than 90 degrees in the air. Make sure you do not arch your back while doing this exercise. Your tailbone should be heavy and your core tight.

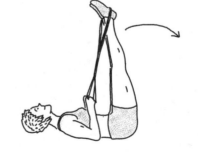

3. Slowly lower your legs until your feet are a few inches from the ground for a count of 10.

4. Then raise your legs with control for a count of 10 to return to the starting position.

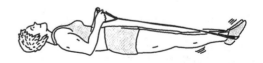

5. Repeat the up and down movement until muscle failure. Then try to lift your legs for a count of 10.

Don't wait to start exercising. In fact, I recommend you start moving now. Get your resistance bands, if you do not already have them, and start these high-intensity workouts right away. Getting your body used to moving before you start making changes in your diet will set you up for the shifts you are about to make.

RULES OF THE GAME

To give you an idea of the way you will be eating in Phase 1 of the Spice Diet, I have summarized the fundamentals of my plan in these rules:

1. Do not eat food that comes in a box, a can, a bag, or in most jars. Processed and prepared food is designed to make you want more. You will be eating whole, fresh food.
2. Refined sugar is taboo. On food labels, if any ingredient ends with "-ose," it is a sugar.
3. Stay away from food that is white or made with white flour, such as potatoes, rice, pasta, bread, cookies, and cake. These types of simple carbohydrates convert to sugar very quickly in your body.
4. Do not drink calories, unless you're having a nutritious smoothie. No soft drinks, juice drinks, beer, alcohol, sugary sports drinks, vitamin-infused water, or creamy coffee concoctions. A glass of wine when you are in Phase 2 is fine.
5. Drink more water, preferably filtered. It will fill you up and flush you out.
6. Foods and drinks labeled "diet" or "sugar free" are not for you. Artificial sweeteners make you hungry.
7. No fried foods. Aside from the calories, fast foods are fried in polyunsaturated oils and partially hydrogenated oil, which are not good for you.
8. Eat lean protein. Chicken, fish, eggs, and reduced-fat dairy products are the way to go. You should limit red meat to two or three times a week.
9. Have olive oil every day—it's liquid gold! I also recommend organic coconut oil and grapeseed oil.
10. Eliminate artificial food additives such as preservatives, coloring, and MSG, which are found in most condiments, ready-made sauces, and soups. Highly processed meat, including cold cuts, sausage, and hot dogs, also fall into this category.

11. Eat more fresh fruits and vegetables, preferably organic ones. The fiber they provide supports weight loss. Limit your fruit consumption to three servings a day, and avoid high-sugar fruits like grapes, which are sugar bombs.

12. Do not eat after dinner. Studies have shown that when you eat after dinner, your body is more likely to store those calories as fat, because you are generally less active at night and do not burn those calories for energy. The other downside to snacking at night is that people tend to select highly palatable, sweet, and salty food when they are tired and have been careful all day. Eating your largest meal at lunch can help you to lose weight. You have more of a chance to burn lunchtime calories than those you eat at dinner.

Although this list might seem limiting, the Spice Diet is not about deprivation. You are making positive changes that will help you fuel your body and lose weight at the same time. You will not be hungry. The food you will be eating is blissfully satisfying.

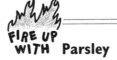

FIRE UP WITH Parsley

Parsley is a lot more than a bright green garnish you see everywhere. It has a host of health benefits and can support your weight loss efforts. Parsley aids digestion for more efficient food processing, which will also boost your metabolism.

Parsley has a mild diuretic effect. You can kick-start your diet by drinking parsley tea. It's a snap to make. Just boil water and pour 1 cup over ¼ cup of chopped fresh parsley. Let it steep for 5 minutes. You can add lemon for flavor.

The diuretic effect of the parsley will reduce water retention, and you will lose weight, at least temporarily. That can be encouraging when you start the program.

There is no end to the uses of parsley. Use the herb on salads and vegetables, and in soups, sauces, marinades, and salad dressings.

Out with the Junk

Before you start Phase 1, I recommend clearing out your kitchen cabinets, refrigerator, and freezer and getting rid of the food you will not be eating. You do not need to make it easy to cheat—and who needs temptation right at hand? In the following chapter, I will tempt you with the delicious foods you will be eating to replace the junk. In the meantime, get rid of:

All oils (except olive oil, raw organic coconut oil, and grapeseed oil)
Anything in a can except organic beans
Barbecue sauces
Bread
Butter
Cake mixes
Cakes
Canned soup
Chips
Cookies
Crackers
Diet anything, including diet sodas
Flavored rice mixes
Frozen prepared meals
Fruit juices
Half-and-half
Heavy cream
Ice cream
Jellies and jams with sugar
Ketchup
Low-calorie ice pops
Mac-and-cheese mix
Margarine
Muffins
Pancake mix
Pasta
Pretzels
Processed cheese
Processed meat
Relishes
Rolls
Salad dressings
Sauces in jars
Soda
Sugar
Sugar substitutes
Sugary sports drinks
Sweetened yogurt
Taco shells
Waffles
White flour
White rice
Whole milk

If you want to lose weight and be healthy, you will not be eating these foods. If you feel bad about throwing away food, give it to friends and family, but know that you are not doing them a favor. You can give any nonperishable, unopened food to charity.

If your partner or children are not ready to change their eating habits, clear a shelf in your kitchen cabinet and your refrigerator for yourself so that you can isolate your food from theirs. Your family will see you change day by day, and they will certainly enjoy the delicious meals you will be preparing. When they smell and taste what's coming from the kitchen, they may become converts to your new way of eating. After all, there's nothing like a home-cooked meal. It won't be long before your family sees the value—and pleasure—of eating the Spice Diet way.

Update Your Spice Rack

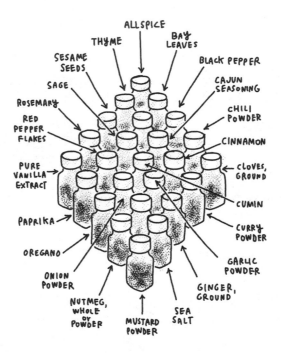

You didn't think you could start Phase 1 without updating and refreshing your spice rack, did you? I have narrowed down all the possibilities to the absolute essential spices you will need to have on hand. If you like, you can also purchase fresh versions of many of these spices, but consider this your start-up spice rack:

Allspice

Bay leaves

Black pepper

Cajun seasoning

Chili powder

Cinnamon

Cloves, ground

Cumin

Curry powder

Garlic powder

Ginger, ground

Sea salt

Mustard powder

Nutmeg, whole or ground

Onion powder

Oregano

Paprika, sweet and smoked

Vanilla extract (pure)

Red pepper flakes

Rosemary

Sage

Sesame seeds

Thyme

Target Your Date to Begin

Pick a date when you want to start changing your eating habits for good. Look at your calendar and find a two-week period without too many social commitments, travel plans, or holidays. Being at a dinner party, traveling, or celebrating as you begin Phase 1 could be very challenging. Find a quiet time in your schedule when you can take control of what you eat. Many people like to begin on a weekend, because they have more time to shop for food and prepare some meals and snacks in advance.

I went cold turkey when I made the decision to change my life. I was gung-ho and ready to dive right in. If you feel the same way, go right ahead. If you prefer weaning yourself off the foods to which you are addicted, it's fine to ease into the Spice Diet. I suggest cutting back gradually a week or two before you start Phase 1. Gradual withdrawal might make doing without your trigger foods less of a shock. Once you start Phase 1, you will be saying good-bye to those foods.

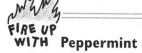

FIRE UP WITH Peppermint

Studies have shown that the smell of peppermint can make you eat less. A cup of steaming peppermint tea can be a wonderful substitute for a sweet dessert. Peppermint is known to:

- Suppress appetite.
- Reduce tension, which can cause bingeing.
- Aid digestion and ease constipation.
- Speed up metabolism.

In addition to tea, I love to use mint in salads and smoothies and with vegetables and fruit. I even make a pesto sauce with mint.

Portion Control

We live in such a time of abundance that portions have become supersized, which has led to routine overeating. In addition to loading foods with hidden, high-calorie ingredients, most restaurants serve at least twice the amount of food you should be eating. Even if what you are eating is healthy, the amount of some foods you consume has to be limited. Portion control is a big part of changing your relationship with the food you eat, and one of the key tenets of mindful eating is controlling the amount of food you eat. To eyeball how much you are eating, here are some basic guidelines for estimating portion size:

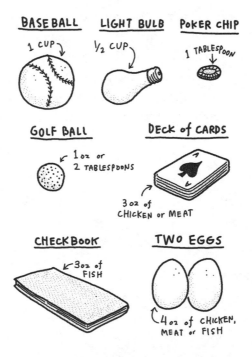

BASEBALL   1 CUP

LIGHT BULB   1/2 CUP

POKER CHIP   1 TABLESPOON

GOLF BALL   1 oz or 2 TABLESPOONS

DECK of CARDS   3 oz of CHICKEN or MEAT

CHECKBOOK   3 oz of FISH

TWO EGGS   4 oz of CHICKEN, MEAT or FISH

- 1 cup = a baseball
- ¾ cup = a tennis ball
- ½ cup = a lightbulb or computer mouse
- ¼ cup = 1 egg
- 1 ounce or 2 tablespoons = a golf ball or Ping-Pong ball
- 1 tablespoon = a poker chip
- 1 teaspoon = 1 die

Recommended amounts of certain foods look like this:

- 3 ounces of cooked chicken or meat = a deck of cards
- 4 ounces of chicken or meat = 2 eggs
- 3-ounce fish fillet = a checkbook
- 4 ounces of fish = 2 eggs
- 1 ounce of cheese = tube of lip balm or standard pink eraser
- 1 ounce of 70% cacao dark chocolate = box of dental floss
- 2 tablespoons salad dressing = a golf ball
- 1 tablespoon nut butter = a poker chip

It's easy to sit with a bowl of nuts and eat the whole thing before you know it, or to slather tons of almond butter on a celery stick. You have to be aware of how much of these foods you are eating, because they stop being healthy alternatives if eaten in too great a quantity. These are reasonable portions for some snacks and other foods:

- ¼ cup (about a handful) of raw nuts and seeds:
  - 23 almonds
  - 18 medium cashews
  - 12 hazelnuts
  - 8 Brazil nuts
  - 12 macadamia nuts
  - 15 pecan halves
  - 14 walnut halves
  - 49 pistachios
- Extra-virgin olive oil: 2 tablespoons
- Apples: 4 ounces (the size of a baseball)
- Limit pineapple to ½ cup

- Only have 1 banana a day
- For Phase 2—cooked quinoa, brown rice, gluten-free pasta: ½ cup as a side dish (the size of a lightbulb), 1 cup as a main course (the size of a baseball)
- For Phase 2—sweet potato: 3 ounces = a computer mouse
- Eat as many vegetables, melons, and berries as you want.

The key is to learn to know when you have had enough to eat and are no longer hungry. When you eat mindfully, you'll see that it does not take that much to fill you up.

Great Expectations

In the beginning, you might find it helpful to create a daily log to record your progress. You will be recording how many calories you consume with each meal and snack, how much water you are drinking each day, and how much sleep you got the night before. This sort of information can be recorded on your phone or computer. What is more important is to write in a journal about how you are experiencing your attempt at transformation. You should identify your Diet Personality (or Personalities—see page 38) as well as your triggers and food cravings. As you progress through Phase 1, write about your highs and lows, any food cravings you might experience, any stumbles, any changes in your energy and mood, and any challenges you experience. This record will show you what works for you and what doesn't and help you identify trends in your personal habits.

You should be noting for each week:

Diet Personality (or Personalities—see page 38)
Personal Narrative (note the potential source of your diet personality and how it manifests in your life)
How I Committed (your overall plan for how you will address your addiction and overcome it)
How I Felt (include physical and emotional reactions during the week)
Weight Loss Expectations (how much you hope to lose during the week), including BMI, waist, and waist-to-height ratio
Actual Loss (your weight loss for the week)

This is a page out of my own journal:

Phase I—Week I, Day I
Diet Personality: The Sweet Tooth
Personal Narrative (Week I):

I have always had an affinity for sweets. I believe it started with my grandma being the best home baker ever. She made something sweet at lunch and dinner. My first experience of baking was when I competed against her at our church bake-off. She always saw the cook or chef in me. She taught me her famous chocolate pound cake recipe, which I baked to compete against her signature brownies. Since many others and I were addicted to these fudgy nuggets of goodness, I knew I did not stand a chance. Grandma won and, much to my surprise, I came in second place, beating out more than fifteen entries.

My grandparents watched over us after school when I was in grammar and elementary school. Along with the chocolate sensations, I remember being treated to the world's best banana milk shakes. My sweet tooth carried with me through my life and grew into an insatiable addiction.

How I Committed (Week I):

My plan is to shift my palate to appreciate the spices that capture the flavor experience of sweetness. For example, instead of consuming cookies and my favorite key lime pie all the time, I plan to focus on sweets like fruit, fruit purees, and fresh sorbets. If I can significantly reduce my love for sweets, anyone can.

How I Felt (Week I):

I was edgy about going through the day without my sugar fix. I found myself thinking about sweet indulgences, even though I wasn't hungry. I acknowledged those thoughts, took a few deep breaths, and let them drift away. It happened ten or twelve times a day, but I stuck with it. I distracted myself by planning what I would eat for the next three days, thinking about an activity that would get me moving during the weekend, or going for a brief walk every time a craving hit, if only to the restroom or to get a glass of water. I was excited about my ability to stop those cravings cold, though I didn't know how long my resistance would last. I took a long look at that graduation photo and resolved that those days were over.

One of my friends tried to persuade me to skip my workout and go out for pizza. I wasn't tempted, but my friend persisted. It upset me that he wouldn't take no for an answer, especially after I told him I was cutting back. If this keeps happening, I can't spend time with him. I don't need a friend undermining my good intentions.

Weight Loss Expectations Week 1: (2–2.5 pounds)
Actual Loss: 2.5 pounds

You should record temptations, victories, emotional experiences, discouragement, frustrations, and optimism. Having a record of what you are going through emotionally will give you an understanding of what you need to do to stay on track.

Now you have prepared yourself mentally and strategically to start Phase 1. All the steps you have taken so far will give you the solid support you need to stick with your efforts to transform your life. At this point, you should be charged up and ready to take the leap to embrace change and reclaim your health and well-being.

7

THE SPICE DIET PLAN PHASE I: MAKING NICE WITH SPICE

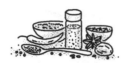

You are committing to following the guidelines of Phase 1 for thirty days. During this time, you will begin to form healthy eating habits. Significant change happens when you make a radical shift in what you eat each day, as it did for me. Keep in mind that this is not a quick-fix, magic-bullet weight loss plan. I'm not promising that this will be easy by any stretch of the imagination, but if you're willing to put in the work and dedication to change your habits and commit to immediate change, the architected spice blends and ingredients in my recipes—and those you will learn to create on your own—will propel you toward your goal.

You can expect to lose up to ten pounds in the first month eating *The Spice Diet* way, which is a healthy and sustainable loss of about 2.5 pounds a week. If your goal is to lose additional weight, you can stick with Phase 1 beyond the initial thirty days until you are close to your dream weight.

More important for the long term, as you enjoy the food on the plan, you will be retraining your taste buds to respond to flavor combinations that are more subtle than the sugar/salt/fat blast of the junk food you are used to eating. Not only do my recipes deliver megawatt flavor, but the functional blends of spices will work with your system to improve your health and metabolism from the inside. As the Fire Up sidebars have noted, the spices I use are medically proven to lower blood sugar, reduce inflammation, settle your digestive system, and provide a host of health benefits along with powerhouse flavor.

It's time to fight and be the master of your fate. Put the power of spices to work for you.

PLAN AHEAD

When I committed myself to battling my weight for the long term, I knew from experience that the best way for me to take control of my eating was to plan my meals and snacks in advance. I was realistic enough to know I'd get into trouble if I was left scrounging around for something to eat when I was hungry. Talk about mindless eating! It helps when you control the foods that are available to eat in your immediate environment, and planning ahead will help you from being tempted to eat too much of the wrong things. At the beginning, not having too much choice will help you to stick with the program. It may seem limiting, but it works, and you will thank me later.

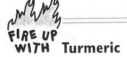

FIRE UP WITH Turmeric

Research has found that when animals are fed curcumin, the active ingredient in turmeric, they lose more fat than those on the same diet without curcumin. Turmeric has been shown to:

- Reduce inflammation, a leading factor in obesity.
- Reduce fat accumulations.
- Boost metabolism.

Use this brightly colored yellow spice as a seasoning in stews, soups, vegetables, and nuts. It's a real fat buster!

As you start Phase 1 of the Spice Diet, I have included two weeks of daily meal plans in this chapter to take the guesswork out of what to eat. In preparing for Phase 1, you have already gotten rid of the foods you should avoid eating. Before I get to the nitty-gritty details of Phase 1, let's get clear on what you should and should not eat in Phase 1.

THE HAVES AND HAVE NOTS OF *THE SPICE DIET*

I have compiled lists of some of my top choices for foods you should eliminate from your diet, some you should limit, and the clean food you can enjoy guiltlessly. I call these lists the "Haves and Have Nots of Healthy Eating." If you follow these food choice dos and don'ts and make the healthy core foods part of your lifestyle, I promise you will see change. You will lose weight, feel better than you ever thought you could, and glow with super-energy. Eating nutritious meals will not only fuel your body, but will lift your spirits as well.

Changing what you eat is a small price to pay for such great benefits. The recipes in *The Spice Diet* will deliver extraordinary flavor, mouth-watering aromas, decadent mouthfeel, and crunchy textures in the healthy meals you will be making.

Stay Away

The foods in the following list are toxic for you. It's time for a Dear John letter to these substances in your life. It's that simple. When you are tempted to eat anything on the list or food that contains one of these ingredients, remind yourself that they are poison for you and are obstacles on your path to a slimmer, more radiant, and healthier you.

Alcohol (beer and liquor)—Don't curse me out under your breath!

Artificial sweeteners

Baked goods—breads, muffins, cakes, cookies, crackers—made with white flour

Canned fruits with added sugar

Canned soups

Canned vegetables

Fatty fried foods

Frozen meals

High-fat meats

High-fructose corn syrup

Hydrogenated oils

Ice cream

Junk snack foods (candy, salty chips, microwavable popcorn, pretzels)

Pastas made with white flour

Peanut butter

Processed cheese (cheese singles, cheese that comes in a can, cheese spreads)

Processed foods that come in a box, can, or bag

Processed meat (canned meats, hot dogs, bologna, salami, chicken nuggets)

Refried beans

Salad dressings in a bottle

Salted or smoked nuts and seeds

Soda or soft drinks

Sugar-free products

Sugary fruit drinks

Sugary sports drinks

Whole milk

Artificial Sweeteners Make You Hungry

Although sugar substitutes contain no calories, they can contribute to weight problems. Artificial sweeteners can interfere with your body's natural regulating processes. Artificial sweeteners trick your body, which judges the number of calories in what you eat by how it tastes. When you drink a diet soda, for example, your taste buds communicate to your brain that energy is coming in in the form of sugar. Since there are no calories in the soda, your body does not get the expected fuel. When the expected calories don't arrive, signals are sent to your brain that your body needs to be fed, leaving you hungry.

Sugar substitutes trick your body in another way. They are 200 to 13,000 times as sweet as sugar. The "feel good" hormones in your brain, such as the endorphin dopamine, respond in kind to such an extremely strong signal. As more endorphins are produced, your pleasure increases, which can lead you to eat more. As you know, the taste of sweetness can be addictive. You are getting a sugar high without the calories of sugar, which leaves your body craving the expected energy. "Diet" foods, most of which use artificial sweeteners, set off a vicious cycle that results in increased hunger and the increased food intake that follows.

Indulge

The foods on the list that follows are at the core of the Spice Diet. Make sure you stock your pantry with these staples and have plenty of fresh items on hand. You will be surprised by the variety of delicious, satisfying meals you can create with these ingredients. While you are following the meal plans, my advice is to buy three to five days of ingredients at a time.

Vegetables

Arugula

Asparagus

Avocados

Beans, dried or organic canned (black beans, kidney beans, pinto beans, cannellini beans, garbanzo beans)

Beets

Bell peppers

Bok choy

Broccoli

Brussels sprouts

Cabbage

Carrots

Cauliflower

Chiles (jalapeños, Thai chiles, habaneros, ghost peppers, chipotle peppers, poblano peppers, Fresno peppers)

Cucumbers

Fennel

Garlic

Ginger

Green beans

Herbs (fresh)

Kale

Lentils

Lettuces and greens (Boston, bibb, butter, endive, oak leaf, and romaine lettuces, collard greens, Swiss chard, rainbow chard, endive, radicchio)

Mushrooms

Onions (Spanish, red, sweet, scallions, ramps, leeks, shallots)

Parsnips

Popcorn, air-popped

Radishes

Spinach

Squash (acorn, butternut, calabaza, delicate, hubard, kabocha, patty pan, pumpkin, spaghetti, yellow zucchini)

Tomatoes

Watercress

Fruit

Apple

Applesauce, all natural, unsweetened

Berries (strawberries, blueberries, raspberries, blackberries, goji)

Citrus (lemon, lime, grapefruit, blood orange, orange, tangerine, clementine)

Melons (cantaloupe, Crenshaw, honeydew, watermelon)

Peach

Plum

Pear

Protein

Eggs

Fresh fish loaded with omega 3 fatty acids (salmon, mackerel, sardines, anchovies, lake trout, herring, snapper, cod, halibut, catfish)

Lean meat (pork tenderloin, filet mignon, flank steak, skinless chicken and turkey.

Protein powder, 100% plant based

Shellfish (shrimp, clams, oysters, octopus, squid, mussels, conch, crab)

Tuna (albacore, canned in water)

Oils

Coconut oil, 100% organic

Extra virgin olive oil

Grapeseed oil

Beverages

Coconut milk, light and unsweetened

Coconut water, unsweetened

Fresh vegetable and fruit juices, no sugar added. Limit fruit juices made from sweet fruit, including apples and tropical fruit to twice a week. It is better to eat the whole raw fruit.

Dairy

Milk (skim, 1%, and 2%)

Yogurt, low-fat

Nutmilks (almond and cashew), unsweetened

Condiments

Apple cider vinegar

Cocoa powder, unsweetened

Flavored vinegars

Mustard

Only in Moderation

These foods should not be eaten every day, but if you have them every now and then, it should not be a problem. I recommend limiting your consumption to once or twice a week, as long as they don't put you over your calorie limit in each phase.

If you cannot get through a day without coffee, do not be alarmed to see coffee on this list. Recent studies have shown that moderating your coffee intake can boost weight loss. Animal studies have shown that drinking five or six cups of coffee a day caused increased fat storage and insulin resistance. On the other hand, drinking coffee in moderation, which means three cups or fewer per day, can reduce blood pressure, and prevent weight gain. The researchers believe that too much coffee might hinder the body's ability to use and process fat. You can get by on three cups a day, can't you? Maybe your dependence on coffee is an addiction you need to break. One other point, instead of whole milk, cream, or half and half, you should use only a little skim milk or unsweetened almond or cashew milk in your coffee; and avoid nondairy creamers or other flavored additives. Rich coffee concoctions will add too many calories to your daily intake. You might want to try using flavored coffee beans to satisfy your taste buds.

All-natural frozen fruit sorbets
Coffee—no more than 3 cups a day
Dark chocolate (70% cacao)
Dried fruit (dates, figs, apricots, raisins, cranberries, currants, cherries)
Honey
Mozzarella cheese
Nut and seed butters (sunflower, cashew, and almond)
Parmigiano Reggiano cheese
Pecorino Romano cheese
Pure maple syrup
Red and white wine
Tropical fruits (pineapples, mangoes, bananas)

HEALTHY SUBSTITUTES

After reading the "Have and Have Not" lists, you might be puzzled about how you are going to cook when some ingredients you use all the time are in the "Have Not" category. The fact is that there are healthy substitutes for just about everything. Some replacements might surprise you. I have collected a number of substitutes for simple carbs, sugar, fat, and salt as well as baking ingredients. Vegans, who do not eat dairy, refined flour products, refined sugar, meat, and fish, developed many of the substitutions. If you feel limited by the "have nots," these solutions will open your eyes to a wide variety of possibilities.

Replacing Simple Carbs

Whole wheat for refined flour: Whole wheat flour takes longer to digest, and refined white flour is like eating sugar.

Brown rice for white rice: White rice is refined, removing the nutritious outer shell of the grain. Brown rice retains the husk and bran layers, providing lots of fiber and other nutrients.

"Zoodles" for pasta: You have most likely seen devices advertised on TV for cutting spiral strips from vegetables. Replacing pasta with strips of zucchini or other veggies creates guilt-free pasta. You can find vegetable "noodles" pre-prepared in some grocery stores and markets.

Spaghetti squash for pasta: Just scrape the inside of a roasted spaghetti squash into strands with a fork and you have a delicious pasta substitute.

Cauliflower or turnip mash for mashed potatoes: If you use spices and herbs for flavor or a little olive oil on steamed or roasted cauliflower and turnips and mash, you won't believe you are not eating potatoes with these mashed vegetables.

Grated steamed cauliflower for rice: I love to make cauliflower "fried rice." The textures are very similar.

Quinoa for couscous: Quinoa is a whole grain that is a complete protein. Couscous is made from processed white flour. Is there even a choice?

Nuts for croutons: Why eat toasted bread when you can substitute nutritious nuts for the crunch factor in your salad?

Ground flaxseeds for bread crumbs: Crushing flaxseeds or using flax meal (ground flaxseeds) is a low-carb substitute for bread crumbs.

Almond meal for bread crumbs: Ground almonds will brown just as bread crumbs do.

Rolled oats for bread crumbs: Try seasoning your rolled oats with any spice blend for great flavor.

Replacing Sugar:

Stevia for sugar: Now that you are off artificial sweeteners, try stevia, which is a natural sweetener made from the stevia plant. Liquid stevia can be three hundred times sweeter than sugar, so follow the instructions for use carefully. Powdered stevia is available that can be substituted for the same amount of sugar. Unless otherwise noted on the packaging, you can make a 1:1 substitution.

Cacao nibs for chocolate chips: Nibs are minimally processed crushed cacao beans. They are an excellent source of antioxidants, iron, and magnesium. A lot of sugar is added in the process of converting nibs to chocolate, so get back to the basics and still get the flavor of chocolate.

Cinnamon for cream and sugar in coffee: Just a sprinkle of cinnamon can complement the flavor of coffee so well you will not miss the sugar.

Unsweetened iced tea for juice: Fruit juice can be loaded with sugar. There are so many flavors of tea available now. Make your own and keep a pitcher in the refrigerator. Don't forget the fresh mint!

Pureed fruit: I use pureed fruit in my smoothies and also as a sauce. There is no need to rely on sugary syrups.

Replacing Fat:

Unsweetened almond or coconut milk for dairy milk: Obviously, there is no animal fat in almond milk. I use it in smoothies all the time. You can use almond or coconut milk as you would use milk from cows.

Banana "ice cream" for ice cream: I have an extravagantly delicious recipe for banana "ice cream" on page 183. To make simple banana ice cream, all you have to do is freeze bananas and then puree them. A dollop can add creaminess to a smoothie.

Coconut milk for heavy cream in soups and stews: If you want a creamy texture without having to rely on fat, try coconut milk. It's delicious and heart-healthy.

Greek yogurt for sour cream: I use Greek yogurt to top my chili and Mexican food these days, and don't miss the sour cream at all.

Greek yogurt for mayonnaise: Just add some spice and herbs and a squeeze of lemon juice to make a terrific spread.

Mashed avocado for mayonnaise: As you know, in my previous life I could never have enough mayonnaise. Now I use mashed avocado, which is packed with healthy fats, and the texture is great.

Ground poultry for ground beef: When you want to cut down on saturated fat, use ground turkey or chicken. Because the fat content is lower than beef, ground poultry can get dry in cooking. Adding a little chicken stock will keep it moist.

White-meat skinless poultry for dark-meat poultry: There is a reason people fight over the juicy drumstick! The fact is, dark meat has a lot of fat. White meat is higher in protein and iron.

Bison for beef: Look for bison in your market. It's low in fat and has more B vitamins than beef.

Prosciutto for bacon: Bacon is one of the most loved flavors. Prosciutto is a better choice, because it is aged and not processed.

Sauté in chicken or vegetable stock rather than oil: You don't have to use oil to sauté. The broth won't brown what you are cooking as well as oil, but it does boost flavor and lightens up the dish.

Replacing Salt:

Herbs or citrus juice for salt: Using herbs and spices can outdo the flavor that salt gives food. Citrus juice can make food sparkle in your mouth.

Garlic powder for salt: Garlic can provide a ton of flavor to what you are cooking. I use granulated garlic, a different product that you can also find in the spice aisle as well.

Homemade salad dressing for bottled: Bottled salad dressing is full of sugar, salt, chemicals, and preservatives. Making your own dressing will not only save you money, but will taste so much better.

Replacing Baking Ingredients:

Pureed black beans for flour: Drain and rinse a 15-ounce can of organic beans and puree them. The can is equivalent to a cup of flour. Pureed beans are a terrific swap for flour in brownies.

Vanilla extract for sugar: The rule of thumb when you are using vanilla extract as a sugar substitute is to cut the amount of sugar in half and add a teaspoon of vanilla. If the recipe already calls for vanilla, use the 1 teaspoon in addition to the amount called for. Substituting vanilla extract is a good way to cut back on your use of sugar.

Mashed bananas for baking fat: Creamy mashed bananas are a great thickening agent. One cup mashed banana = 1 cup fat.

Unsweetened applesauce for sugar: Applesauce substitutes for sugar in a 1:1 ratio. Because applesauce is practically liquid, reduce the amount of liquid in the recipe by ¼ cup.

Unsweetened applesauce for butter: This substitution works well in muffins and sweet breads. To start, only replace half the fat with applesauce and use butter or oil for the other half. Experiment to find the right balance.

Avocado puree for butter: Avocado and butter have close to the same consistency at room temperature and they are both fats. Avocado works well in recipes with dark chocolate, like brownies. One cup pureed avocado = 1 cup (2 sticks) butter.

Prune puree for butter: To make a butter substitute that works for dark baked goods, combine ¾ cup dried prunes with ¼ cup boiling water and let soak for 15 minutes. Puree in a blender or food processor.

Chia seeds for butter: You may have seen chia seeds used for pudding. When combined with fluids, chia seeds produce a gel. As a butter substitute, combine 1 tablespoon chia seeds with ½ cup plus 1 tablespoon water. Let the mixture stand for 15 minutes. The gel is a good stand-in for fat when you are baking. I don't suggest totally replacing fat with chia gel. Use half the fat called for in the recipe and the equivalent amount of chia gel.

Chia seeds for eggs: Those chia seeds certainly are versatile. Mix 1 tablespoon chia seeds with 1 cup water. Let the mixture sit for 15 minutes; the resulting mixture is equivalent to 1 egg. It's not a good idea to replace both butter and eggs with a chia substitute in the same recipe.

Flax meal for eggs: Mix 1 tablespoon flax meal (ground flaxseeds) with 3 tablespoons warm water and whisk until combined. Refrigerate the mixture for 5 to 10 minutes; the resulting mixture is equivalent to 1 egg.

Buying, Using, and Storing Spices and Herbs

Spices and herbs are at the heart of your new way of eating, so I want to give you some background on the dry-versus-fresh question. Some people think that fresh herbs are always the best option, but that is not necessarily the case. Many spices, including pepper, allspice, and cloves, come into the height of their flavor only after drying, because enzymes are activated in the drying process. Most spices you will be using are grown in the tropics, which would make them difficult to get fresh. The fact is that the majority of spices are at their best when dried. Fresh spices get their flavor and aroma from volatile oils and oleoresins in the cell structure of the plant. Over time, the oils evaporate and the spice loses its flavor and aroma.

Remember that dusty spice rack in my mother's kitchen? The spices had been sitting around for so long that the contents of those jars were probably useless. Don't buy large quantities, unless you use a particular spice regularly, because the flavors of a spice dissipate and flatten over time. Make a point to not keep spices after the use-by date. You'll be sacrificing flavor if you do, and flavor is what spices are all about. Your spice rack should be placed out of direct sunlight. Some dried spices and herbs, such as parsley or chives, have a very delicate cell structure. That is why spices should be kept in the pantry, away from heat, light, and humidity.

To test dried herbs for freshness, put a few leaves in the palm of your hand and rub them with your thumb. By the time the leaves turn to powder, the warmth from your hand and the rubbing should release the aroma. If what you smell is strawlike or musty, that spice is over. Throw it away. If you are using a whole spice or herb, break off a piece and grate it. Give it the sniff test. Again, if the aroma does not capture the essence of the spice, the punch of the flavor has been reduced. If you want great flavor, use spices that are at their peak.

When you are buying dried herbs and spices, pay attention to the packaging. Stay away from cardboard boxes or low-barrier plastics, which oxygen can permeate, causing the spice to degrade. As pleasant as the experience can be, I avoid buying spices that can be scooped from bins, because the spices may have been exposed to bacteria, bugs, and a lot of air. Spices are best stored in jars with airtight lids. High-barrier resealable plastic packaging, which gases and moisture cannot permeate, can extend the life of dried spices and herbs, especially if you squeeze the air out before resealing the package.

Do not shake or pour dried spices and herbs directly from the jar over a steaming saucepan. If you do, you risk steam condensation around the opening of the container. The moisture can cause mold to form and make the spice oxidize.

Fresh herbs that are soft such as parsley, tarragon, dill, basil, chervil, mint, and cilantro can last a week in the refrigerator. After washing the herbs, put them in a glass with an inch of water at the bottom and cover the leaves with a plastic bag. You can leave the herbs on the counter in a glass with an inch of water if you change the water every three days or so.

It can be frustrating to buy fresh herbs for a recipe that requires only a tablespoon of the chopped herb. There is no need to waste perfectly good herbs or have them go bad in your refrigerator. There is an easy way to freeze herbs for future use. Chop soft herbs finely. Fill an ice cube tray with the chopped herb until each section is about two-thirds full. Add water to cover the chopped herb and freeze. When the cubes are completely frozen, remove the herb cubes, put them in a plastic bag, and store the bag in the freezer. The herb will be available whenever you need it. For storing herbs with hard stems, like rosemary, wrap the stems in foil and place the packet into a resealable plastic bag. Freeze the bag until you need the herbs.

If you are lucky enough to be able to grow your own herbs, you can harvest them and dry them yourself when your plants are producing too quickly for you to use them up or the season is about to end. Herbs you dry at home will be far more fragrant and colorful than commercially dried herbs. You do not have to invest in a dehydrator to preserve your herbs for future use. You can air-dry your herbs or dry them in the oven or microwave. Air-drying is most effective with low-moisture herbs such as dill, rosemary, oregano, thyme, sage, and marjoram. Herbs containing more moisture, including mint, basil, and chives, dry better in the oven or microwave.

When you are planning to dry some herbs from the garden, cut the herb stems mid-morning, after the dew has dried, to achieve maximum flavor. Remove any wilted, yellowing, or sickly leaves. If rinsing is required, make sure you pat the herbs dry very well. You can dry herbs by spreading fresh cut stems on a parchment-lined baking sheet and leaving the stems to dry at room temperature. It's a good idea to turn the herb stems every few days to ensure even drying. Or you can tie the herbs in small bundles of five to ten stems with string or a rubber band and hang them upside down to dry indoors. Find a spot out of direct sunlight, because too much sun can cause flavor loss and color fading. Either way, your herbs might be dried and ready to store in as little as a week. It depends on the level of humidity.

To dry herbs in the oven, place the herb, seeds, or stems in one layer on a baking sheet. Put the herbs in an oven set on low heat (lower than 180°F) with the door open for two to four hours. The herbs are ready when the leaves are crisp, dry, and crumble easily. Oven-dried herbs will lose some of their flavor because they cook a bit while you are drying them. You may need to use a little more of these oven-dried garden herbs when you cook with them.

You can also nuke the leaves in a microwave. In fact, using the microwave is a great way to preserve flavor and color. Microwaves specifically target water as they are heating. We've all had the experience of nuking something for too long and having it become completely dehydrated and turn into a rock. This works in your favor with herbs. Microwaving an herb can make the water content evaporate quickly and leave flavor compounds and pigments behind. And the process is fast. Simply remove the leaves from the stems and spread them in a single layer on two paper towels, which have been placed on a microwavable dish. Do not used recycled paper toweling, because recycled paper sometimes contains bits of metal that can explode or cause a fire. Cover the leaves with another paper towel or a clean dishtowel. If you are drying hard herbs, put the herbs in the microwave and cook them for about a minute, then do a few twenty-second bursts until the leaves are dry. Delicate or soft herbs will take about forty seconds followed by twenty-second bursts until completely dry.

Whether you air-dry, oven-dry, or microwave your herbs, the test for when the herbs are dry is the same: When the leaves crumble easily and small stems break when they are bent, the herbs are properly dried. If they are not dry enough, leathery or soft herbs will develop mold, so you want to be sure the moisture is removed. Strip the dried leaves from the stem and keep them whole to store in airtight containers. Crush the leaves when you are ready to use them. The dried herbs should last a year if stored correctly (see page 122). Taking care of your herbs and spices will ensure that they enhance your cooking with the layers of flavor you want.

You Can Thrive without the "Have Nots"

When I was about to start Phase I of the Spice Diet, I was nervous about dropping simple carbohydrates and processed sugar from my diet. I usually put two teaspoons of sugar in my coffee, drank at least three cans of soda a day, no meal was complete without bread, and then there was dessert. Before I took the leap, I tried to wean myself from my addictions. I wasn't very successful. I started drinking unsweetened coffee, but my sugar cravings kicked in, and I ended up eating more cookies and candy. Since gradually cutting back wasn't working, I knew I had to go cold turkey.

I studied Judson's food Haves and Have Nots and jumped right into Phase I. I made a promise to myself to stick to the guidelines. I decided to start on the weekend so that I could take it easy and focus on cooking and planning snacks and meals for the following week. My husband offered to plan a weekend of fun for the kids. He was delighted to have some time alone with them. So off they went.

During that weekend, I learned what withdrawing from drugs must be like. As the day went on, I was grouchy and developed a roaring headache. My energy took a nosedive. I had stocked up for the weekend, so I was able to stay in bed or lie on the couch most of the day. I figured it was a good time to binge watch a couple of shows I had missed. I also treated myself to a lot of old movies. All I could think about was sweets. The cravings intensified. I felt hollow, but I knew it would pass. When my family came home that evening, they found me in bed with the covers over my head.

I felt better the next morning. I was still edgy and had mild flu-like symptoms, but I knew I had been through the worst of it. If I made it through the previous day, I believed I could do it again. I did some cooking, and the food tasted great. I'm not saying that I didn't crave a muffin and a rich coffee drink, but I didn't feel as if I could eat the couch. I was so grateful to my husband for giving me the space to go through my withdrawal from sweets alone. I would have been a bear to be with.

I was still a bit shaky on Monday, but I had been through two days without sugar and the symptoms were much less intense. The distraction of work was a good thing. At the end of the third day, I was over the hump. It takes time to change habits, but the physical cravings had substantially subsided. After a couple of weeks, I had beaten it—at least for the near future. If I lost the battle and had to go through it again, I would know what to expect. Of course, the thought of another "lost weekend" made me increase my resolve. If I was going to lose a weekend, I wanted it to be a "get away from it all" treat. Sunning my slim self on a tropical beach in a tiny bikini was where I wanted to be!

—*Melanie D.*

PHASE I GUIDELINES

As you begin the Spice Diet, it's important to keep track of the calories you are consuming. It might seem old-fashioned, but believe me, it works. It's so easy to underestimate your caloric intake. Knowing the caloric value of what you eat is an important part of getting your weight loss program off to a good start and transforming your diet forever. The recipes in chapters 9 and 10 have calorie counts to make the task easier.

PHASE I CALORIE RANGE

These are the acceptable daily caloric ranges for women and men. If you keep your caloric intake at midrange, you will definitely lose weight.

Woman: 1,000 to 1,600 calories a day = 1,300 optimum total calories a day
Men: 1,200 to 1,700 calories a day = 1,500 optimum total calories a day

> For optimal weight loss, try to keep your daily food intake to the guide-
> lines I have suggested. Don't forget to count everything you eat. Don't
> cheat, however strong the impulse. You want an honest assessment of what
> it takes for you to lose weight.

Keeping track of the calories you consume is so much easier than it used to be. There are many free sites online and apps for your phone. The calorie trackers that get the best reviews include My Fitness Pal, Lose It!, Fat Secret, Cron-O-Meter, Spark People, and Diet Hero. If you download an app for your phone, you can record your calories when you eat your meals so you don't have to remember what you've eaten in order to record it later. Make keeping track of what you eat a habit.

Guilt-Free Snacks

You will not starve on the Spice Diet. Plan to have a midmorning snack and another midafternoon. Making a habit of drinking water is also part of the plan. Increasing your water consumption is a good way to suppress hunger. Although the amount of water you should consume is not one-size-fits-all, on average, men should consume thirteen 8-ounce glasses of liquid a day and women should consume nine 8-ounce glasses.

Building snacks into your day will keep your blood sugar level from dipping between meals and will satisfy your taste buds. Healthy snacks are important in your daily diet to keep your metabolism going throughout the day, which helps to manage your weight and balance your diet. Snacking with good-for-you choices can:

- Prevent cravings and overeating.
- Help to maintain mental and physical energy throughout the day.
- Aid with portion control at dinner, when most people tend to over-indulge in food.

I often eat a small portion of leftovers as a snack. Having a few healthy snack items on hand will make Phase 1 a breeze. Pack up a few non-perishables in suggested portions and take them to work. You can keep others in the refrigerator packaged as individual snacks. Some snacks you can enjoy in moderation that can satisfy your taste for something sweet, crunchy, salty, or creamy include:

Almond or cashew butter (1 tablespoon) on celery, slices of banana, apple, or pear

Almonds or cashews, raw, unsalted (6 to 12)

Apple, pear, plum, peach, nectarine (medium)

Avocado (half) with 1 tablespoon vinaigrette

Broth or clear soup (1 cup)

Cantaloupe, honeydew, or watermelon cubes (1 cup)

Cheese (1 ounce cheddar, feta, Swiss, Gouda, cottage cheese, Parmigiano Reggiano) on apple slices

Chef Judson's "Peach Cobbler" Power Bar and Citrus Protein Bar (see pages 167 and 202)

Crudités (carrot spears, celery, bell pepper slices, mushrooms, broccoli, cauliflower) dipped in:

- bean dip (2 to 4 tablespoons)
- guacamole (2 to 3 tablespoons)
- hummus (2 to 4 tablespoons)
- roasted red pepper dip (2 to 4 tablespoons)
- salsa (2 to 4 tablespoons)

Fat-free or 1% cottage cheese/ricotta cheese (4 ounces) with herbs and spices

Fat-free or light cream cheese (2 tablespoons)

Hard-boiled egg

Kale chips (homemade; see page 164)

Marinated artichoke hearts

Olives

Orange or grapefruit (small)

Peanuts, raw, unsalted

Pickled vegetables

Pistachios raw, unsalted

Plain nonfat Greek yogurt (6 ounces) with fresh fruit or homemade fruit
  puree added

Roasted vegetables

Roll-ups—a lettuce leaf or a slice of turkey filled with hummus, carrots,
  or leftover vegetables

Slice of turkey or roast chicken

Strawberries, blueberries, blackberries, or raspberries, or a mix (1 cup)

Sunflower or pumpkin seeds, raw, unsalted (½ ounce)

Vegetable juice (fresh)

Walnuts raw, unsalted

TWO WEEKS OF MEAL PLANS FOR PHASE I

Following are meal plans for the first two weeks of Phase 1 to assure you that
you will not go hungry when you eat the Spice Diet way. Instead, you will look
forward to every snack and meal, which will be bursting with powerhouse
flavor. The recipes for the Phase 1 Meal Plans can be found in chapter 9. Feel
free to shift meals and snacks from one day to another. You might be too busy
to prepare a suggested recipe on a particular day so rather than go off the
plan, substitute another recipe or one of your own. Go right ahead and customize your meals as long as you stay within the caloric restrictions and follow the Haves and Have Nots lists (see page 113). You will be more successful
if you tailor the menu to your tastes and needs.

There is great variety in the meal plans, but you might find that you like
one snack so much you want to eat it every day, or you might repeat a favorite meal often. If that is the case, you can make a big batch of the recipe so
that it's ready for you when you want it. For example, if you love the bone
broth, you can double or triple the recipe and freeze the extra broth in individual servings. You can make a big pot of chili and eat it all week or freeze
the extra to eat in the future. The only limitation is that you should try to
avoid eating beef more than twice a week.

I love leftovers and have built them into the menus. You can recycle
dinner as your lunch a day or two later, as I have done a few times in the
meal plans. Look over the menus for the week. Make your shopping list

and buy what you will be eating in the next three or four days. The pleasure of anticipation will make your transformation easier, and food cravings will fade as you fully satisfy your taste buds. If you have a plan and look forward to what you are going to eat, you will be much less likely to go astray.

Of course, I have included a number of indulgent desserts. I suggest you plan to have desserts two or three times a week. I always save mine for the weekend, but you might choose to finish a meal with something sweet after a hectic weekday. When you have your two or three desserts a week is up to you.

Although you can start Phase 1 at any time, most people want to start out fresh and begin something new on a Monday. This works well, because you can prepare some items in advance during the weekend, such as bone broth, Quiche without the Carbs individual frittatas, seasoned nuts, and Chef Judson's "Peach Cobbler" Power Bar so that you have a supply on hand for the busy week ahead. I have designed the menus with that in mind.

When I suggest using a spice blend, you can replace it with any blend you would like to try. If you have not yet made the spice blend I recommend, feel free to use a commercial seasoning such as Cajun, Italian, or curry powder, as long as the blend contains little to no salt or sugar. Remember this important fact: If salt or sugar is among the first ingredients listed on the label, put that bottle down. Ingredients are listed by quantity in decreasing order. The first ingredient is the predominant ingredient in the product. You will undermine your efforts if your intake of salt and sugar increases, so read labels carefully.

You are about to make a very big change in your life. The Spice Diet will reward you by giving you a new way to approach food that will light up the pleasure center in your brain as it boosts your health and well-being. Enjoy! You have a lifetime of pleasurable eating ahead.

Day 1

Breakfast	Scrumptious Savory Scramble (page 149)
Snack	Basic Bone Broth (page 169)
Lunch	Lemon-Pepper Shrimp and Kale Salad (page 162)
Snack	Sweet-and-Sour Dill Pickle Cashews (page 163; 18 nuts)

| Dinner | Golden BBQ Chicken with Southern Collard Greens (pages 177 and 179) |
| Dessert | Summer Day Sorbet (page 182) |

Day 2

Breakfast	1 cup nonfat Greek yogurt with fresh strawberries, blueberries, or raspberries or a mixture of berries, sprinkled with unsweetened coconut flakes.
Snack	Sliced apple with 1 tablespoon almond butter.
Lunch	Beef (80% lean), turkey, chicken, veggie, or fish burger with lettuce, tomato, sliced onion, and avocado. Don't be tempted to use mayo; instead, swap in a quality Dijon mustard or pesto.
Snack	Popcorn seasoned with the spice blend of your choice (pages 226–252).
Dinner	Tuna Poke Bowl (page 159) or any grilled, baked, or broiled fish with my pecan crust (page 210) with mixed roasted vegetables with spice blend of your choice.

Day 3

Breakfast	Any herb and vegetable combination two-egg omelet.
Snack	Chef Judson's "Peach Cobbler" Power Bar (page 167).
Lunch	Leftover BBQ chicken with a cucumber dill salad with nonfat Greek yogurt dressing.
Snack	Sweet-and-Sour Dill Pickle Cashews (18 nuts; page 163).
Dinner	Rustic Chicken Sausage Stew (page 174).

Day 4

Breakfast	Quiche without the Carbs Individual Frittata (page 148).
Snack	Fresh cut veggies with Honey-Fig Hummus (page 165).
Lunch	The Ultimate Tuna Salad (page 195) on a bed of lettuce, wrapped in a lettuce leaf, or on tomato rounds.
Snack	Basic Bone Broth (page 169).

Dinner   Lip-Smacking Chicken Wings (page 158) with Sesame-
            Ginger Kale Chips (page 164).
Dessert   Tropical Sorbet (page 183).

Day 5

Breakfast   Everything but the Kitchen Sink Green Drink
            (page 156).
Snack   Mixed olives in brine with Moroccan Spice Blend
            (page 241).
Lunch   Leftover Lip-Smacking Chicken Wings with Sesame-
            Ginger Kale Chips (page 164).
Snack   Raw unsalted pecans.
Dinner   Broiled or grilled steak with garlic cauliflower mash and
            steamed green beans with almonds, tarragon, and a touch
            of olive oil.

Day 6

Breakfast   Guilt-free Pancakes (page 152).
Snack   1 piece of fruit, your choice.
Lunch   Chipotle Chicken and Black Bean Soup (page 171).
Snack   1 low-fat string cheese or 1 ounce reduced-fat cheese.
Dinner   Quick-and-Easy Jamaican Red Snapper Escovitch
            (page 176) with steamed vegetable of your choice with
            lemon.
Dessert   Buttery Macadamia Nut "Ice Cream" (page 183).

Day 7

Breakfast   Bright Eye Juice (page 154).
Snack   Celery with 1 tablespoon almond butter.
Lunch   Coconut Squash Soup (page 170) with a spinach and
            mushroom salad.
Snack   Sesame-Ginger Kale Chips (page 164).
Dinner   Chinese Sweet-and-Spicy Chicken Kebobs with Easy Relish
            (page 172) and steamed broccoli.

Day 8

Breakfast	Diced melon and mint mixed with plain nonfat Greek yogurt, sprinkled with 1 tablespoon chopped pecans or any nut of your choice.
Snack	Cajun Brussels Sprout Chips (page 165).
Lunch	Leftover Chipotle Chicken and Black Bean Soup (page 171).
Snack	Popcorn with spice blend of your choice (page 226–252).
Dinner	Broiled shrimp with Chesapeake Bay Crab and Seafood Spice Blend (page 233) with steamed or roasted asparagus with balsamic vinegar and a crumbled hard-boiled egg.

Day 9

Breakfast	One-egg Southwest omelet with peppers, onions, tomatoes, and/or salsa with 1 turkey sausage link.
Snack	Chef Judson's "Peach Cobbler" Power Bar (page 167).
Lunch	Leftover broiled shrimp with avocado and tomato.
Snack	Pistachio Nuts (49 nuts) baked in oil with the Jamaican Me Crazy Jerk Spice Blend (page 237).
Dinner	Salmon Cobb salad (4-ounce piece of broiled or grilled salmon, 2 tablespoons chopped avocado, 1 strip of low-sodium turkey bacon, cooked and crumbled, a hard-boiled egg, and up to 2 tablespoons low-fat dressing).

Day 10

Breakfast	Everything but the Kitchen Sink Green Drink (page 156).
Snack	Up to 2 cups watermelon cubes with mint.
Lunch	Romaine lettuce roll-ups with hummus, asparagus, carrots, cucumber spears, and thinly sliced low-fat, low-sodium, all-natural turkey, roast beef, or ham.
Snack	Guacamole with fresh cut veggies.
Dinner	Effortless Thai Fried "Rice" (page 157).

Day 11

Breakfast	Quiche without the Carbs Individual Frittata (page 148).
Snack	Popcorn with your favorite spice blend (page 226–252).

Lunch	Leftover Effortless Thai Fried "Rice" (page 157).
Snack	Honey-Fig Hummus (page 165) with raw vegetables.
Dinner	Grilled or broiled salmon, cod, red snapper, halibut, or tilapia with spice blend of your choice (pages 226–252) and Basic Cauliflower Rice (page 179).

Day 12

Breakfast	Two eggs, any style, with 2 turkey sausage links.
Snack	A medium orange, pear, banana, or apple with 10 almonds.
Lunch	Beef (80% lean), turkey, chicken, fish, or veggie burger topped with slices of avocado, tomato, and red onion with mustard yogurt sauce (see page 224).
Snack	Chai Pumpkin Smoothie (page 153).
Dinner	Golden BBQ Chicken with Charred Moroccan Broccolini (page 176).

Day 13

Breakfast	Savory Turkey Bacon, Cheddar, and Cauliflower Pancakes (page 151).
Snack	Sweet-and-Sour Dill Pickle Cashews (18 nuts; page 163).
Lunch	Coconut Squash Soup (page 170) with a mixed green salad.
Snack	Pecan-Maple Shake (page 155).
Dinner	Rustic Chicken Sausage Stew (page 174) prepared using leftover Golden BBQ Chicken (page 177) from the previous night.

Day 14

Breakfast	Spice Diet Smoked Salmon Benedict (page 150).
Snack	Chef Judson's "Peach Cobbler" Power Bar (page 167).
Lunch	South-of-the-Border Grilled Corn Bisque (page 203).
Snack	Brussels Sprout Chips (page 165) with Blueberry Pop (page 156).
Dinner	Grilled or broiled chicken breasts seasoned with the spice blend of your choice (make extra for leftovers) and Grilled Peach and Kale Salad (page 180).
Dessert	Tropical Sorbet (page 183).

I've created this menu plan to give you a sense of how varied and delicious your life can be even while losing weight. After two weeks, you can repeat these menus or plan your own meals for the next two weeks of Phase 1. Feel free to mix it up for variety. At the end of the month, stepping on the scale should make you smile. You will be on your way to achieving your goals.

If you want to lose more weight, you can stay on Phase 1 indefinitely. When you hit a plateau, as most everyone does at some point, exercise more. You might try adding some aerobic exercise to your day. That would be any movement that gets your heart pumping. You don't have to run on a treadmill forever to get results. Interval training, which is another form of high-intensity exercise, can help you when your weight feels stuck. It's called 10-20-30 training.

10-20-30 TRAINING TO BREAK THROUGH PLATEAUS

The *New York Times* reported that researchers in Denmark have come up with a new approach to high-intensity interval training in a way that makes it less challenging. A complete 10-20-30 session lasts twelve minutes! This is how it is done:

- Walk, ride a bike, work out on an elliptical or rowing machine gently for 30 seconds.
- Speed up to a moderate pace for 20 seconds.
- Sprint or work out as hard as you can for 10 seconds.
- Rest for 2 minutes by walking slowly or standing.
- Repeat sequence a total of 4 times.

That's a total of forty seconds of hard work—less than a minute—for the entire session. It doesn't get easier than that! When you have built up your stamina, you can repeat five times instead of four.

High-intensity interval training (HIIT) should not be done on consecutive days, so you will be doing the 10-20-30 training three or four times a week in addition to your band workouts. Doing this interval training for twelve minutes every other day will rev up your metabolism and make you feel great. Adding interval training to your high-intensity band workouts will boost your fitness, build muscle, and turn your body into a calorie-burning machine.

MOVING ON

Congratulations! Once you have completed the first thirty days of your new life, snap a picture of yourself and put it next to your starting photo on your vision board or wherever you have your before photo. Can you see a difference? Are you looking better already? Is it easier to zip up your jeans? Check your BMI, waist circumference, and weight-to-height ratio and compare your new numbers with your starting measures.

You may decide to stay on Phase 1 for an additional thirty days to take off more weight. Once you have been preparing Spice Diet foods for thirty days, you should be feeling more at home in the kitchen and ready to get more creative with your spices and ingredients. When you want to add more variety to any dish, you can experiment more with the spice blends in chapter 11. After following Phase 1, you have formed healthier eating habits and are well on your way to reprogramming your taste buds.

When you are ready to move to Phase 2, you should be close to the weight you want to be. Now is the time to refine the habits you have developed and to shift into maintenance mode. In Phase 2, your goals are to keep the weight off, feel great, and live a life full of flavor.

8

THE SPICE DIET PLAN PHASE 2: MASTERING HEALTHY HABITS LONG TERM

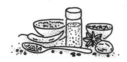

Phase 2 is the way to eat for the rest of your life to maintain the weight you have lost during Phase 1. You will concentrate on the healthy habits you began forming in the first phase. You can continue to lose weight gradually during Phase 2, but the more rapid results of Phase 1 are always available to you at any time you want to return to it.

In Phase 2 your caloric intake increases from Phase 1. Continue to keep track of what you are eating until you adjust to your new calorie range. It is easy to underestimate the calorie content of what you are eating.

PHASE 2 CALORIE RANGE

The ideal number of calories you will be eating in Phase 2 is a bit higher than that of Phase 1.

Women: 1,600 to 1,800 calories a day = 1,700 optimum total calories a day
Men: 2,200 to 2,400 calories a day = 2,300 optimum total calories a day

In this phase, it is important not to exceed these caloric limits, because that is when the weight will come back. If you keep within these ranges, you will continue to lose weight but at a slower pace than during Phase 1.

You can now add some carbs and grains to what you eat, including whole wheat pasta, sweet potato, brown rice, wild rice, quinoa, and other grains. As a side dish, your portion size will be ½ cup, the size of a computer mouse or a lightbulb. If you are eating the carb as the base for an entire meal, the portion size is 1 cup, the size of a baseball.

You can also add a slice of whole wheat bread each day. I recommend Ezekiel bread, which is not a brand of bread but a type of bread. Reference is made to Ezekiel bread in the Bible:

Take also unto thee Wheat, and Barley, and beans, and lentils, and millet, and Spelt, and put them in one vessel, and make bread of it.
—*Ezekiel 4:9*

Today, Ezekiel bread uses the same recipe. The bread is made from organic sprouted whole grains, including wheat, millet, spelt, barley, and the legumes soybeans and lentils, the same ingredients as mentioned in the Bible verse. Added sugar is not in the ingredients of Ezekiel bread, as it is in most commercial whole wheat breads. When the grains and legumes are sprouted and combined, a complete protein, containing all nine essential amino acids, is created that closely parallels the protein found in milk and eggs. In fact, the protein quality is so high that Ezekiel bread contains an additional eighteen amino acids present from vegetable sources. Another plus is that the bread is very high in fiber, which fills you up and is slow to digest, keeping you full longer. Ezekiel bread has an appealing nutty flavor and provides a nutritional bonanza. When you have a choice, go with Ezekiel bread. You will not be consuming empty calories.

The recipes in Phase 2, which you will find in chapter 10, are not as calorie restrictive as those in Phase 1. They fall within the recommended range to prevent you from regaining the weight you lost in Phase 1. This next level of recipes will expand your already wide variety of breakfast, lunch, dinner, snack, dessert, and drink choices. I keep my desserts to twice a week and usually save them for the weekends!

I know that maintaining a healthy lifestyle long-term is not easy. Indulging in convenience foods, sugary desserts, and salty snacks now and then as well as eating out can eventually allow your old habits to creep back. It's happened to me. I was determined to break out of the yo-yo diet cycle as my weight spiraled up. I was going to be rigid about what I ate. I came to understand that no one is perfect. Backsliding happens to everyone. Do not be hard on yourself if you have a temporary setback. If you do fall off the wagon, the Spice Diet is there to lift you up. By following the "haves and have nots" of food choices (see page 113) and making healthier foods the core of your diet, you will be able to rebound, pick yourself up, and get back to clean eating. Here are some general guidelines for maintaining your weight loss:

- If you notice that your weight has gone up five pounds, return to Phase 1. You don't want your weight gain to be like a runaway train.
- If you find cravings sneaking back, return to Phase 1 to reinforce the good habits you are forming.
- If you blow it big time, remember it's only a single meal, dessert, or snack. If you have overeaten, you can make a correction the next time you eat.
- If your weight loss is slowing down, exercise more and return to Phase 1.
- When you have reached your desired weight, follow the 80/20 rule, which I will explain in detail in chapter 12. The general rule of thumb is that if you eat well 80 percent of the time, you should be able to keep you weight under control.
- When you indulge, do so mindfully. You have to make a conscious decision to eat something from the "have not" list or to chow down on supersized portions. You have to choose going off track occasionally. If unchecked, mindless eating will get you back to where you started.

MEAL PLANS FOR PHASE 2

I have put together two weeks of meal plans to give you an idea of how to incorporate some carbs into your diet without going overboard. You are welcome to substitute your own recipes for any of my suggestions. Just keep in mind that you should add carbs and grains carefully and watch the calorie count. By now, you should be feeling comfortable cooking with spices and turning out great meals that fill you up and nourish your body.

Just as I did for the meal plans for Phase 1, in Phase 2 I have gone for variety, incorporated leftovers into the plan, and added desserts on the weekends. You might love a single snack or recipe and repeat it a number of times in a week. Repetition can save you preparation time. You can double or triple many of the recipes and freeze them for future meals. You can also return to recipes you liked from Phase 1. There is nothing wrong with a healthy habit, but you don't want to get bored by eating the same meal again and again. The nature of the Spice Diet is to avoid boredom by packing in flavor and variety. So even if you are in love with a specific recipe, change it up now and then. Experience the richness that spice can bring into your life.

At this stage, try experimenting with the flavor profiles in chapter 11. From Jamaican Me Crazy Jerk Blend to Nuts 4 Almond Coconut Crust Blend to Fiesta Spice Blend, you will find twenty-five spice combos that will add "foodgasmic" flavor to the food you prepare.

Day 1

Breakfast	Quiche without the Carbs Individual Frittata (page 148) made with your own veggie and spice combination
Snack	Chef Judson's Citrus Protein Bar (page 202)
Lunch	Chicken Caesar Salad—Hold the Anchovies (page 196)
Snack	Candied Chickpeas (page 200)
Dinner	Salmon Quinoa Bowl (page 197)

Day 2

Breakfast	"Granola" Oatmeal (page 189)
Snack	The Kale-leidoscope Green Drink (page 193)
Lunch	Leftover Salmon Quinoa Bowl (page 197)
Snack	Caramelized Shallot and Spinach Dip (page 198) with raw or roasted veggies
Dinner	Honey-Lemon Baked Chicken (page 207) with Asparagus Mélange (page 213)

Day 3

Breakfast	Banana-Citrus Yogurt (page 191)
Snack	Apple slices with almond butter
Lunch	Ultimate Tuna Salad (page 195) on top of a bed of mixed spring greens

Snack	Basic Bone Broth (page 169) You may have some frozen on hand that you made in Phase 1; otherwise, make a fresh batch. Sipping bone broth is good for you.
Dinner	New Orleans Pecan-Crusted Catfish (page 210) with Maple-Roasted Sweet Potatoes (page 212).

Day 4

Breakfast	Omelet made with leftover Asparagus Mélange (page 213)
Snack	Chef Judson's Citrus Protein Bar (page 202)
Lunch	Leftover Honey-Lemon Baked Chicken (page 207) with Quick-Pickled Green Beans (page 200)
Snack	Aloha Soda (page 193) with 10 cashews
Dinner	Chipotle Chicken and Black Bean Soup (page 171) with any mixed green and vegetable salad

Day 5

Breakfast	Almond "PB&J" Protein Smoothie (page 192)
Snack	The Kale-leidoscope Green Drink (page 193)
Lunch	Beef, turkey, chicken, fish, or veggie burger, seasoned with the spice blend of your choice (pages 226–252) and topped with slices of red onion, avocado, and tomato
Snack	Chef Judson's Citrus Protein Bar (page 202)
Dinner	Baked or grilled fish of your choice with Spiced Kale and Coconut Quinoa Stir-Fry (page 214)

Day 6

Breakfast	Lemon-Blueberry Pancakes with Sweet-and-Spicy Syrup (page 189)
Snack	Celery with a tablespoon of almond butter
Lunch	Veggie Taquitos (page 194) with salsa and guacamole
Snack	Leftover Caramelized Shallots and Spinach Dip (page 198) with raw veggies
Dinner	One-Pot-Wonder Seafood Stew (page 205) with roasted vegetables
Dessert	Chocolate Banana Bites (page 217)

Day 7

Breakfast	Scrumptious Savory Scramble (page 149) with 2 strips of turkey bacon
Snack	1 cup nonfat Greek yogurt with a sprinkle of cocoa and sliced almonds
Lunch	Leftover Chipotle Chicken and Black Bean Soup (page 171)
Snack	Popcorn with the spice blend of your choice (pages 226–252)
Dinner	Grandpa's Vegetarian Chili (page 208) with Basic Cauliflower Rice (page 179)
Dessert	Decadent Peanut Butter Cup "Ice Cream" (page 219)

Day 8

Breakfast	Omelet made with leftover Grandpa's Vegetarian Chili (page 208)
Snack	Big Red Juice (page 192)
Lunch	Lettuce roll-up with thin slices of turkey, roast beef, or ham with hummus, carrots, spinach, slices of pepper
Snack	Popcorn seasoned with your favorite spice blend (pages 226–252)
Dinner	Comfort Meat Loaf (page 206) with Crispy Cauliflower Bites (page 199) and Quick-Pickled Green Beans (page 200)

Day 9

Breakfast	Banana-Citrus Yogurt (page 191)
Snack	Chef Judson's Citrus Protein Bar (page 202)
Lunch	Leftover Comfort Meat Loaf (page 206) with a mixed salad
Snack	Leftover Crispy Cauliflower Bites (page 199)
Dinner	Thai Shrimp Red Curry Soup (page 204) with Basic Cauliflower Rice (page 179)

Day 10

Breakfast	Quiche without the Carbs Individual Frittata (page 148)
Snack	Basic Bone Broth (page 169)
Lunch	Chef salad with thin strips of turkey, ham, and low-fat Swiss cheese, and sunflower seeds

| Snack | Strawberries with black pepper, mint, and balsamic vinegar |
| Dinner | Lip-Smacking Chicken Wings (page 158) with Sesame-Ginger Kale Chips (page 164) |

Day 11

Breakfast	"Granola" Oatmeal (page 189)
Snack	A piece of your favorite fruit
Lunch	Leftover Lip-Smacking Chicken Wings (page 158)
Snack	1 low-fat string cheese or 1 ounce reduced-fat cheese with pistachios
Dinner	Broiled or baked fish of your choice with sweet potato crumble and as many roasted veggies of your choice as you like

Day 12

Breakfast	Quiche without the Carbs Individual Frittata (page 148)
Snack	Leftover roasted veggies
Lunch	Waldorf salad with diced apple, dried cranberries or raisins, walnuts, lemon juice, and 2 tablespoons nonfat Greek yogurt on a bed of lettuce
Snack	Caramelized Shallot Spinach Dip (page 198) with raw veggies
Dinner	Broiled or grilled steak with Spiced Kale and Coconut Quinoa Stir-Fry (page 214)

Day 13

Breakfast	Lemon-Blueberry Pancakes with Sweet-and-Spicy Syrup (page 189)
Snack	Chef Judson's Citrus Protein Bar (page 202)
Lunch	Beef, turkey, chicken, veggie, or fish burger with lettuce, onion, tomato, with Quick-Pickled Green Beans (page 200)
Snack	Mixed olives with a little olive oil and the spice blend of your choice (pages 226–252)
Dinner	Steve Harvey's Favorite Cajun Lobster Mac and Cheese (page 211) with a side salad

Day 14

Breakfast	Spice Diet Smoked Salmon Benedict (page 150)
Snack	18 cashews seasoned with the spice blend of your choice (pages 226–252)
Lunch	Spinach salad with mushrooms, 1 strip of turkey bacon, hard-boiled egg, and avocado
Snack	Candied Chickpeas (page 200)
Dinner	"Zoodles" and Creamy Roasted Tomato Sauce (page 175)
Dessert	Earl Grey–Infused Lemon Granita (page 216) with 1 Grandma's Carrot Cake Oatmeal Cookie (page 218)

The following two chapters contain seventy-two recipes, which will convince you that you can prepare delicious meals in your own kitchen that are more satisfying than takeout or most restaurant food. These recipes will convince you that being a home cook is fun, not drudgery. Hand-choosing the freshest, best ingredients, seasoning those ingredients for maximum flavor, and assembling meals that are a perfect balance of flavor and texture—the entire process is a pleasure. Not only will you enjoy what comes out of your kitchen, but seeing the smiles of your guests and family will also confirm that you have created a peak pleasure experience with healthy food. The aromas alone are enough to entice people to your table to enjoy your "diet" food. So roll up your sleeves and head for the kitchen!

9

POWERHOUSE FLAVOR RECIPES
FOR PHASE I

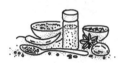

From Guilt-Free Pancakes to Pecan-Maple Shake, from Lip-Smacking Chicken Wings to Sweet-and-Sour Dill Pickle Cashews, from Golden BBQ Chicken to Hazelnut Dark Chocolate Truffles, my mouth-watering recipes will show you that eating well does not require deprivation. This chapter will give you concrete ways to make healthy choices a part of your every-day eating routine. Your family will love these recipes and probably won't realize you have made major adjustments to their diet.

Please do not be put off by what might seem like long lists of ingredi-ents. You are becoming an architect of flavor and constructing layered flavor takes many building blocks. Knowing how busy we all are, the recipes them-selves are easy to prepare.

The core of the Spice Diet is to make the healthy food you are eating as appealing as possible. I want you to look over the list of recipes for Phase 1 and think, "You mean I can eat that when I'm trying to lose weight?" Yes, you can! I have designed these recipes to work with the caloric restrictions of Phase 1.

I have also taken into consideration medically driven diet issues in creat-ing my Powerhouse Flavor Recipes. Though only some of the recipes are vegetarian or vegan, the food you will be eating will promote your health.

The illustrations that follow are icons that represent the benefits of eating the Spice Diet way:

 Immunity Building

 High Protein

 Cholesterol Reduction

 Low Sodium

 Diabetic Friendly

 Omega-3 Rich

 Heart Healthy

 Vegetarian and Vegan

POWERHOUSE RECIPES

Breakfast

Quiche without the Carbs Individual Frittata (page 148)
Scrumptious Savory Scramble (page 149)
Spice Diet Smoked Salmon Benedict (page 150)
Savory Turkey Bacon, Cheddar, and Cauliflower Pancakes (page 151)
Guilt-Free Pancakes (page 152)

Green Drinks, Juices, and Smoothies

Chai Pumpkin Smoothie (page 153)
Bright Eye Juice (page 154)
Pecan-Maple Shake (page 155)
The Creamy Green Dream (page 155)
Everything but the Kitchen Sink Green Drink (page 156)
Blueberry Pop (page 156)

Lunch

Effortless Thai Fried "Rice" (page 157)
Lip-Smacking Chicken Wings (page 158)
Tuna Poke Bowl (page 159)
Mediterranean Turkey Burger (page 161)

BREAKFAST

Having a delicious, nutritious breakfast has been shown to reduce your hunger pangs throughout the day. Getting into the habit of planning a good breakfast instead of grabbing something on the run is the best way to set yourself up for high energy and a day of healthy eating. My breakfast recipes will give you an idea of the terrific food you will have when you eat the Spice Diet way. You've never been "on a diet" like this before. There is nothing bland or boring about the foods that you will make in your own kitchen. Get ready for an adventure in food!

QUICHE WITHOUT THE CARBS INDIVIDUAL FRITTATA

Serves: 6
Serving size: ⅙ frittata
Calories per serving: 240

Frittatas are making a mighty comeback and make entertaining easy, because you can make a frittata in advance and serve it at room temperature or just warm it up so you won't get stuck in the kitchen. If you make a frittata on the weekend, you will have breakfast ready for the rest of the week.

It's also great to have a supply of frittata "cupcakes" in the freezer—all you have to do is warm one or two up in the microwave for breakfast, lunch, or a snack. To make individual frittatas, simply pour the mixture into a muffin tin lined with paper liners or lightly rubbed with olive oil. Get creative and come up with your own combinations of vegetables and spices for your frittata.

1 Vidalia onion, finely diced	2 handfuls of baby spinach
1 tablespoon balsamic vinegar	1 garlic clove (or more, if you like garlic), mashed
2 tablespoons water	
8 large eggs	1 teaspoon fresh thyme leaves
¼ cup skim milk	1 teaspoon red pepper flakes
10 ounces turkey breakfast sausage, cut into ¼-inch-thick coins	1 cup low-fat cottage cheese

Preheat the oven to 350°F.

In a 10-inch skillet, combine the onion, vinegar, and 2 tablespoons water. Cook over medium heat for 35 to 40 minutes until the onion is caramelized.

Combine the eggs and milk in a bowl and whisk until combined. Add the sausage, spinach, garlic, thyme, caramelized onion, red pepper flakes, and cottage cheese.

Pour the mixture into an oiled cast-iron skillet, a nonstick oven-safe skillet, or an oven-friendly ceramic dish. Keep in mind that a great frittata has a custardlike consistency. Bake for 20 to 30 minutes, depending on size and thickness. Play it safe and check 5 minutes before your frittata is done. Serve slices of the frittata right from the oven or at room temperature.

SCRUMPTIOUS SAVORY SCRAMBLE

Serves: 4
Serving size: ⅔ cup
Calories per serving: 200

Scrambled eggs are my go-to breakfast. And keeping it real, I love them for lunch and dinner as well! The combinations of flavors and textures that you can create are endless. A great tip: Use leftover proteins, veggies, and spice blends to build the ultimate scrambled egg dish. As a major bonus, this super-easy way of cooking eggs is cost efficient and saves on preparation time.

If you are concerned about cholesterol and want to avoid egg yolks, this dish can be made using egg whites. Depending on your taste for heat, you can eliminate the serrano peppers, reduce the amount, or add more.

Juice of ½ lime

1 avocado, diced

2 scallions, thinly sliced (about ⅛ inch thick)

½ serrano pepper, end removed, seeded, and diced small

½ cup heirloom or regular cherry tomatoes, halved

1 teaspoon finely chopped fresh cilantro, plus more for garnish

6 eggs, or 2½ cups egg white equivalent

½ teaspoon olive oil

In a medium bowl, combine the lime juice, avocado, scallions, serrano pepper, tomatoes, and cilantro. Mix and set aside.

In a separate medium bowl, whisk the eggs. In a 10-inch skillet, heat the oil over medium-low heat. Pour the eggs into the skillet. As the eggs begin to set, gently pull them across the pan with a spatula, forming large, soft curds. Cook, pulling, lifting, and folding the eggs, until thickened and no visible liquid egg remains. Remove from the heat and divide among four plates. Top evenly with the avocado salad. Garnish with fresh cilantro. Serve immediately.

SPICE DIET SMOKED SALMON BENEDICT

Serves: 4
Serving size: 1 egg and the spinach and sauce divided evenly
Calories per serving: 241

Although I've put this dish in the breakfast section, you can enjoy it at any meal. I find that if I start out with a hearty meal, my hunger is reduced for the rest of the day. The combination of egg, fish, spinach, and yogurt is a nutritional bonanza.

Reducing preparation time in the kitchen is golden, so buy prewashed baby spinach. Remember that nonfat Greek yogurt is the quintessential substitution for heavy cream, mayonnaise, cream cheese, and other high-fat ingredients that are typically used to add richness to your food.

2 teaspoons olive oil, divided

1 tablespoon thinly sliced or pressed garlic

1 teaspoon fresh lemon juice

10 ounces prewashed baby spinach

4 large eggs

½ pound smoked salmon, thinly sliced

⅛ teaspoon minced fresh dill

½ teaspoon chopped fresh chives

2 tablespoons plain nonfat Greek yogurt

In a skillet, heat 1 teaspoon of the olive oil over medium heat. Add the garlic and cook, stirring, for 1 minute. Add the lemon juice. Stir in the spinach and cook for 2 to 3 minutes, until the spinach has wilted.

In a separate nonstick skillet, heat the remaining 1 teaspoon olive oil. Crack the eggs into the skillet and cook over-easy. (If you don't like over-easy eggs with runny yolks, cook them to your desired doneness.)

Divide the spinach mixture among four plates and top each with an egg. Divide the smoked salmon and fresh herbs among the plates and finish each with ½ tablespoon dollop of yogurt.

SAVORY TURKEY BACON, CHEDDAR, AND CAULIFLOWER PANCAKES

Serves: 3
Serving size: 2 pancakes
Calories per serving: 123 (244 with optional ingredients)

Pancakes made from cauliflower? Just wait until you taste them! Forget about the maple syrup. These savory pancakes will inspire a new appreciation for one of the healthiest foods on earth. The rich supply of health-promoting phytochemicals and anti-inflammatory compounds found in cauliflower helps in the prevention of cancer and heart disease and promotes weight loss.

Riced cauliflower is exceptionally versatile and works as a substitute for simple carbs like rice and flour. You can reduce a head of cauliflower to the size of rice kernels in a food processor or purchase a 12-ounce bag of riced cauliflower from your local grocery store to save time on making it from scratch. It doesn't take much time, so give it a try at least once.

Olive oil cooking spray

1 (12-ounce) bag cauliflower rice, or 1 head cauliflower, cut into florets

1½ teaspoons olive oil

1 teaspoon minced garlic

1 teaspoon finely chopped fresh chives

2 tablespoons chopped scallions

1½ tablespoons almond flour or almond meal

1 egg, beaten

¼ cup shredded low-fat cheddar cheese

3 strips cooked turkey bacon, broken or chopped

⅓ cup honey (optional)

1 tablespoon Sriracha (optional)

Preheat the oven to 400°F. Line a baking sheet with parchment paper and spray the parchment paper with cooking spray.

(If you are using the pre-bagged riced cauliflower, you can skip this step.) Put the cauliflower florets in a food processor and pulse until they break down to the texture of rice. Put the prepared cauliflower in a microwave-safe bowl. Microwave for 2 minutes, until cooked through. Cauliflower is very moist and microwaving cauliflower rice draws out the moisture. Let cool for about 5 minutes, then transfer to a large bowl.

Add the olive oil, garlic, chives, scallions, almond flour, egg, cheddar, and bacon and combine the ingredients with a fork. Form the mixture into 4 to 6 patties and place them on the prepared baking sheet.

Bake for 15 to 20 minutes, or until golden and crispy.

For heightened flavor, in a small bowl, whisk together the honey and Sriracha and drizzle over the pancakes.

GUILT-FREE PANCAKES

Serves: 10
Serving size: 3 small pancakes
Calories per serving: 141

You have probably eliminated pancakes from your diet in your struggle to lose weight. The good news is that you do not have to give up pancakes when you eat the Spice Diet way. This recipe for guilt-free pancakes will satisfy your cravings for the sweet treat.

The banana in this recipe not only acts as a great binder for your pancakes but also is a perfect substitute for added sweeteners. Another tip is to use pure vanilla extract when baking. My grandma always added a little more vanilla than what a recipe called for, and you should, too. You will thank me for this tip.

1½ cups almond flour or almond meal

¼ teaspoon ground nutmeg

1 tablespoon unsweetened cocoa powder (add another tablespoon if you like the dark chocolate flavor)

1 teaspoon baking powder

1 ripe banana, mashed

1 cup unsweetened almond milk

1 tablespoon pure vanilla extract, plus more if needed (you should be able to taste the vanilla in balance with the other flavors)

3 large eggs

Nonstick cooking spray

In a large bowl, combine the almond flour, nutmeg, cocoa powder, and baking powder.

In a separate medium bowl, mash the banana until smooth. Add the almond milk, vanilla, and eggs. Whisk until combined.

Pour the wet ingredients into the dry ingredients and whisk to combine.

Spray a griddle or skillet with nonstick cooking spray and heat over medium-high heat. Ladle batter onto the griddle in circles. Cook on one side for 3 to 4 minutes, or until golden with crispy edges. Flip the pancakes and cook the other side for 2 to 3 minutes. Transfer to a plate and repeat until you have used all the batter.

GREEN DRINKS, JUICES, AND SMOOTHIES

Juices and smoothies are all the rage. It seems that there are juice and smoothie bars on every corner in Chicago—along with the coffee shops. My contributions to the juice craze are in a league of their own. The flavor is incomparable, and, of course, I give a nod to the addition of spices that enhance the taste profile and make the juices and smoothies unique. Try these recipes, and you will not be tempted to buy overly sweet juices and smoothies again!

CHAI PUMPKIN SMOOTHIE

Serves: 2
Serving size: 1½ cup
Calories per serving: 244

This ultra-rich smoothie is a delightful treat—like dessert in a glass. Pumpkin spice is a major flavor of the comfort food category. If pumpkin does not get you excited, you could substitute butternut squash or sweet potato for that ingredient. When you select nondairy milk substitutes, remember to purchase unsweetened varieties. Calorie-wise, it makes a huge difference. Milk made from nuts—almond milk, for example—is naturally sweet.

Seeing an avocado in the ingredients list of a beverage might surprise you. Avocados take on the flavor of other ingredients and make everything creamy and rich. I have substituted dried dates for processed sugar in this recipe. If you didn't know about the substitution, you wouldn't taste the difference.

½ cup pumpkin puree, canned or fresh

2 cups unsweetened almond milk

1 tablespoon fresh orange juice

½ avocado, pitted and peeled

4 Medjool dates, pitted

1 teaspoon pure vanilla extract

1 teaspoon chai spice tea

5 ice cubes

½ teaspoon ground cinnamon

⅛ teaspoon ground nutmeg

Combine all the ingredients in a blender and blend until smooth.

BRIGHT EYE JUICE

Serves: 4
Serving size: 1⅔ cup
Calories per serving: 186

This juice balances the sweetness of carrot and pineapple with the pungency of turmeric. The brilliance of the orange carrot and hot yellow of the turmeric make this delicious juice a treat for your eyes, too.

2 pounds carrots (about 10 medium), chopped

4 cups fresh or frozen cubed pineapple

2 tablespoons ground turmeric

Run the carrots, pineapple, and fresh turmeric through a juicer into a glass. If you are using ground turmeric, add it to the juice and whisk to incorporate.

If you do not have a juicer, simply combine the carrots, pineapple, fresh or ground turmeric, and 1 tablespoon water in a blender and blend until smooth. Strain this mixture through a fine-mesh sieve or a colander lined with cheesecloth to get the pure juice.

PECAN-MAPLE SHAKE

Serves: 1
Serving size: a little more than 1 cup
Calories per serving: 332

This creamy shake delivers powerhouse flavor. It is so rich, you almost need to eat it with a spoon!

I banana

1½ tablespoons coarsely chopped pecans

2 tablespoons instant oatmeal

I cup unsweetened almond milk

I tablespoon pure maple syrup

2 tablespoons nonfat Greek yogurt

½ teaspoon ground cinnamon

Combine all the ingredients in a blender and blend until well combined. Add 2 or 3 ice cubes to the blender with the other ingredients.

THE CREAMY GREEN DREAM

Serves: 1
Serving size: 2 cups
Calories per serving: 175

This refreshing smoothie resembles a tropical frozen drink—without the alcohol. The banana adds creamy sweetness, and the kale is nutrient dense.

I cup unsweetened light coconut milk

½ cup coconut water

I banana

3 kale leaves, hard stems removed

I heaping cup ice cubes

Combine all the ingredients in a blender and blend until smooth. Serve immediately.

EVERYTHING BUT THE KITCHEN SINK GREEN DRINK

Serves: 1
Serving size: 2¼ cup
Calories per serving: 314

Talk about blending flavors—this smoothie is full of fruits, green vegetables, and seeds. As you enjoy the way the drink tastes, you will also get a high-nutrition boost.

- 2 tablespoons raw unsalted pumpkin seeds
- I tablespoon raw unsalted sunflower seeds
- I tablespoon dried cranberries
- I tablespoon chopped dates
- Handful of spinach
- Handful of kale
- ½ red apple, cored
- 1½ cups coconut water

Combine all the ingredients in a blender and blend until smooth. Add 2 or 3 ice cubes to the blender with the other ingredients.

BLUEBERRY POP

Serves: 3
Serving size: 1 cup
Calories per serving: 50

You won't miss your colas and sweet soft drinks after you try this berry-herb soda. If you are not a fan of blueberries, you can replace them with blackberries or any combination of your favorite berries.

- I cup fresh or frozen blueberries or berry of choice
- ¼ cup water
- I tablespoon honey, plus more to taste
- 2 cups sparkling water
- 6 fresh basil leaves

In a blender, combine the blueberries, honey, and water and blend until smooth.

Pour the blueberry mixture into a pitcher, add the sparkling water, and stir in the basil leaves with a spoon. Pour into glasses over ice and get ready to be refreshed.

LUNCH

I know many of you are not in the position to prepare an elaborate lunch every day, but with some advance planning, you can make your lunch on the weekend or the night before and heat it up in the middle of the day. What you make yourself will be so much tastier than what you can buy at takeout places, and you won't be tempted to backslide when tons of menus pass your desk at the office featuring triple-decker sandwiches, chicken wings, bacon cheeseburgers, French fries, and chips.

When your family, friends, and colleagues enjoy the aromas and watch you eat, they will want to have what you're having!

EFFORTLESS THAI FRIED "RICE"

Serves: 4
Serving size: 1¼ cup
Calories per serving: 226

I bet you thought you would never eat fried rice again. Well, I've come up with a recipe that fills the bill. My fried "rice" uses cauliflower rice, which is a delicious substitute for white rice, along with mango and chicken. To save time, you can purchase pre-packaged riced cauliflower from your grocery store.

I use my Thai Spice Blend in this recipe. While you're preparing this dish, you can make a large quantity of the spice blend and store it for future use. Everyone who has tried my fried rice recipe makes it their go-to favorite.

You can make this dish in advance and warm it up when you are ready to enjoy it.

1 teaspoon toasted sesame oil

1 tablespoon chopped garlic

3 dried Thai chiles, or 1 teaspoon red pepper flakes

1½ teaspoons grated fresh ginger

1¼ cups riced cauliflower (see page 179), or 1 (12-ounce) bag cauliflower rice

1 pound boneless, skinless chicken breasts, cut into 1-inch cubes (2 cups)

½ teaspoon Thai Spice Blend (page 240)

1 large egg

2 tablespoons low-sodium soy sauce

½ cup diced mango, juice reserved

¾ cup coarsely chopped red bell pepper

¼ cup fresh basil leaves

¼ cup minced scallions

In a large skillet, combine the sesame oil, garlic, chiles, and ginger. Cook over medium-high heat for 1 to 2 minutes. Add the cauliflower rice and cook for 5 minutes. Transfer to a bowl and set aside.

Season the chicken with the Thai Spice Blend. In the same skillet you used for the rice, cook the chicken over medium-high heat, stirring often, for 7 minutes, or until cooked through.

Return the rice mixture to the skillet with the chicken and stir to combine.

Crack the egg over the contents of the skillet and stir with a fork until the egg is scrambled and fully incorporated.

Add the soy sauce, mango and juice, and bell pepper and cook for 3 minutes, or until the bell pepper is soft.

Combine the basil and scallions in a small bowl. Stir all the ingredients to fully incorporate and garnish with the basil-scallion mixture.

LIP-SMACKING CHICKEN WINGS

Serves: 5
Serving size: 3 wings
Calories per serving: 393

I always pair interesting and cool flavors together in my cooking. The honey-fig sauce you will make for these wings is a perfect example. The recipe is super easy to prepare and full of flavor. Foodies as well as kitchen first-timers all appreciate this delectable dish. It's irresistible!

FOR THE HONEY-FIG SAUCE:

⅓ cup beer

⅓ cup honey

4 or 5 large dried figs

FOR THE CHICKEN:

1 pound chicken wings, cut into winglets, wing tips discarded

2 tablespoons olive oil

1 tablespoon lemon zest

1 teaspoon cracked black pepper

½ teaspoon minced garlic

1 teaspoon finely chopped fresh parsley

Preheat the oven to 400°F. Line a baking sheet with parchment paper.

Make the sauce: Combine the beer, honey, and figs in a small, heavy saucepan. Stir over low heat until the honey dissolves. Increase the heat to medium and simmer until the figs are tender, 5 to 7 minutes.

Remove the sauce from the heat, let cool, and transfer to a blender. Blend the sauce until smooth.

Return the sauce to the pot and heat over medium-high heat, stirring frequently, until thickened, 20 to 25 minutes.

Make the chicken: In a large bowl, combine the chicken wings, 2 tablespoons of the honey-fig sauce, the olive oil, lemon zest, pepper, and garlic. Toss well to coat.

Place the wings on the lined baking sheet and bake for 40 to 45 minutes, or until the skin is crispy and caramelized with sauce. Pour the remaining sauce over the wings and garnish with the parsley before serving. Keep in mind that you can always serve the sauce on the side or add it to the chicken wings for a flavor explosion.

TUNA POKE BOWL

Serves: 1

Serving size: Approx. 2½ cups

Calories per serving: 447

Poke, pronounced "PO-kay," is a traditional Hawaiian dish that features raw fish. Although Hawaiians have been enjoying *poke* for centuries, this salad has recently become very trendy on the mainland. If you are planning to make this recipe, build in marinating time. My recommendation is to marinate the tuna in the *poke* sauce for up to 2 hours, which makes the fish more flavorful and tender. If you are looking to make this a "quick meal," no worries! You can cut the marinating time to 20 minutes. If you prefer not to eat raw fish, you can broil or grill the tuna first to the level of doneness you like.

My recipe calls for cauliflower rice, but you can substitute mixed greens, such as shredded kale, spring mix greens, or baby spinach, for the riced cauliflower.

FOR THE SAUCE:

1 tablespoon low-sodium soy sauce

1 tablespoon toasted sesame oil

Pinch of red pepper flakes

¼ teaspoon finely chopped garlic

2 teaspoons pineapple juice

FOR THE POKE BOWL:

4 ounces ahi tuna, cut into ½-inch cubes

1 cup cauliflower rice (see page 179), or 1 (12-ounce) bag riced cauliflower, microwaved

1 radish, thinly sliced

2 tablespoons matchstick carrots, available packaged at most grocery stores

1 tablespoon marinated seaweed or seaweed salad, available at Asian grocery stores or at the sushi kiosks at many markets

2 tablespoons chopped cucumber

1 tablespoon chopped scallion

½ teaspoon white sesame seeds

Make the sauce: Whisk together all the sauce ingredients in a bowl.

Make the poke bowl: Add the diced tuna to the poke sauce, cover the bowl, and let the tuna marinate in the refrigerator for up to 2 hours.

To assemble, put the cauliflower rice in a chilled serving bowl and toss with the radish, carrots, seaweed salad, and cucumber. Add the marinated tuna in the middle of the vegetables. You don't want to overdo the poke sauce because of sodium, so I recommend not adding additional sauce. Garnish with the scallion and sesame seeds. Serve immediately.

MEDITERRANEAN TURKEY BURGER

Serves: 4

Serving size: 1 patty with salad and dressing divided evenly

Calories per serving: 382

Mediterranean cuisine is certainly popular, because of its healthy attributes and bold flavor! This style of cooking has been known to reduce the risk of developing type 2 diabetes, high blood pressure, and cholesterol. This Mediterranean burger is bursting with fresh ingredients. The pickled salad and yogurt sauce amplify the taste experience. You won't even miss the bun!

FOR THE SALAD:

⅓ cup red wine vinegar

¼ cup half-moon slices red onion

½ cup Roma (plum) tomatoes, cut into 6 wedges each

1 teaspoon chopped fresh oregano

FOR THE TURKEY BURGER:

1½ pounds ground turkey

1 large egg, beaten

¼ cup crumbled low-fat feta cheese

1½ tablespoons olive oil

¼ cup chopped dry-packed sun-dried tomatoes

½ teaspoon dried oregano or Mediterranean Spice Blend (page 242)

½ teaspoon ground black pepper

FOR THE YOGURT SAUCE:

½ cup nonfat Greek yogurt

½ teaspoon finely chopped fresh dill

⅛ teaspoon finely chopped fresh mint

2 tablespoons finely diced cucumber

Preheat the broiler.

Make the salad: In a small bowl, combine the vinegar, onion, tomatoes, and oregano. Set aside for 30 minutes.

Make the turkey burger: In a medium bowl, combine the ground turkey, egg, feta, olive oil, sun-dried tomatoes, oregano, and black pepper. Form into 4- to 5-ounce patties and place on a baking sheet. Broil for 5 to 7 minutes on each side.

Turn the oven temperature to 350°F and bake for an additional 10 minutes to ensure doneness.

Make the yogurt sauce: In a small bowl, combine the yogurt, dill, mint, and cucumber. Stir.

Plate the burgers and divide the salad among them. Top each with a dollop of the yogurt sauce.

LEMON-PEPPER SHRIMP AND KALE SALAD WITH CRISPY SHALLOT VINAIGRETTE

Serves: 5
Serving size: 1 fillet
Calories per serving: 230

Shrimp and kale work well together. The colors and textures make an interesting contrast. This recipe ties those contrasts together with a Creamy Roasted Shallot Vinaigrette. This salad is a perfect light lunch or dinner. Once you taste the creamy dressing, I'm sure you will be tossing many other salads with it.

FOR THE SALAD:

1 bunch kale, rinsed and patted dry

About ⅓ cup chicken stock

1 pound extra-jumbo (16–20 count) shrimp, peeled and deveined

¼ cup dried unsweetened cranberries

2 tablespoons raw unsalted sunflower seeds, toasted

1 tablespoon lemon zest

3 grinds black pepper

FOR THE CREAMY ROASTED SHALLOT VINAIGRETTE DRESSING:

1 garlic clove, pressed

1 shallot

2 tablespoons olive oil

½ cup plain nonfat Greek yogurt

Zest and juice of 1 lemon

1½ teaspoons rice vinegar

1 tablespoon honey

Make the salad: Roll up the kale leaves and cut them crosswise into thin strips. This is called chiffonade.

In a medium saucepan, heat ½ inch of chicken stock over medium-low heat. Add the shrimp and cook for 3 minutes if peeled or 4 minutes if in the shell, or until the flesh is opaque. Drain and set aside. Combine the kale chiffonade, shrimp, cranberries, sunflower seeds, lemon zest, and pepper in a medium bowl.

Make the dressing: In a medium skillet, combine the garlic, shallot, and olive oil. Cook over medium heat, stirring, for 4 minutes.

Transfer the shallot mixture to a blender and add the yogurt, lemon zest, lemon juice, vinegar, and honey. Blend until smooth and creamy.

Pour the dressing over the salad and mix until fully coated. Do not over-dress the salad.

SNACKS AND APPETIZERS

Having healthy snacks on hand will help to take the stress out of changing the way you eat. Knowing you can munch on something delicious that will not put your calorie count through the roof makes a big difference. You are not meant to starve on the Spice Diet. You can take your snacks to the office or bring some in the car when you are running around. Eating a scrumptious portion-controlled snack between meals will keep the hunger pangs away.

SWEET-AND-SOUR DILL PICKLE CASHEWS

Serves: 16
Serving size: 18 cashews
Calories per serving: 157

These spiced cashews are one of my favorite snacks. The Sour Dill Pickle Spice Blend complements the delicate sweetness of the nuts. Cashews are not a waste of calories. They are packed with vitamins, minerals, and antioxidants and have many health benefits, including lowering blood pressure and contributing to heart health.

Keep in mind that an ounce of cashews—that's eighteen medium-size cashews—has 157 calories, so although they are nutritious, you should watch your portions. You can put 1-ounce portions into bags or reusable containers to keep yourself from overindulging. They are so delicious, you might find it hard to stop eating them.

You can use the spice blends in chapter 11 with any nuts you like. Play around. I love Jamaican Jerk Macadamia Nuts—but remember that macadamia nuts are high in calories, so limit your portion to 12 nuts. Just coat the nuts lightly with oil, spread them out on a parchment paper–lined baking sheet, and sprinkle with your choice of seasoning.

1 tablespoon honey

1 teaspoon fresh lime juice

1 teaspoon olive oil

1 teaspoon Sour Dill Pickle Spice Blend (page 232)

2 cups raw unsalted cashews

Preheat the oven to 350°F. Line a rimmed baking sheet with parchment paper.

In a bowl, mix the honey, lime juice, olive oil, and Sour Dill Pickle Spice Blend together. Add the nuts and coat them fully.

Spread the nuts on the lined baking sheet and bake for 10 to 15 minutes.

Serve warm or at room temperature.

Nuts can be stored in an air-tight container in the pantry for 6 to 9 months, in the refrigerator away from strong smelling food up to a year, and in the freezer for 2 years.

SESAME-GINGER KALE CHIPS

Serves: 2

Serving size: 2 cups

Calories per serving: 140

If you enjoy the crunch factor as much as I do, you will consider this recipe heaven-sent. Turning a superfood into a chip is a miraculous transformation! The flavors of sesame, ginger, and honey with a little heat from the pepper flakes create a layered effect that make this snack a stand-out.

1 bunch kale, rinsed and patted dry

1 tablespoon olive oil

2 tablespoons toasted sesame oil

Pinch of red pepper flakes

1 teaspoon low-sodium soy sauce

½ teaspoon granulated garlic

1 tablespoon ground ginger

1 tablespoon honey

Preheat the oven to 350°F. Line a baking sheet with parchment paper.

Stem the kale leaves and tear the leaves into large pieces, roughly 4 inches.

In a large bowl, whisk together the olive and sesame oils, red pepper flakes, soy sauce, garlic, ginger, and honey. Toss the kale with the mixture to coat the leaves.

Arrange the kale leaves in an even layer on the lined baking sheet and bake for 15 minutes. Watch carefully to avoid burning the chips.

HONEY-FIG HUMMUS

Serves: 4
Serving size: ¼ cup hummus
Calories per serving: 203

This sweet and spicy play on traditional hummus pairs and balances the flavor of figs with hot sauce, preferably my signature Chef Blend Hot Sauce, which is available on my website. This flavorful and healthy snack is one of my favorites.

1 (15-ounce) can chickpeas, drained and rinsed

½ cup chopped dried figs, plus more for garnish

2 tablespoons hot sauce

2 tablespoons tahini (sesame paste)

2 garlic cloves

1 tablespoon fresh lemon juice

½ teaspoon sea salt

½ teaspoon ground cumin

1 teaspoon olive oil, for garnish

¼ cup pomegranate seeds, for garnish

1 tablespoon finely chopped fresh parsley, for garnish

Fresh vegetables, for dipping

In a blender or food processor, combine the chickpeas, figs, hot sauce, tahini, garlic, lemon juice, salt, and cumin. Blend until smooth and creamy. You are looking for a thick, dip-like consistency.

Transfer to a dish or bowl and garnish with olive oil, chopped figs, pomegranate seeds, and chopped parsley.

Serve with fresh vegetables.

CAJUN BRUSSELS SPROUT CHIPS

Serves: 4
Serving size: 1 cup
Calories per serving: 85

I must admit, I am addicted to spicy Brussels sprout chips! I call them the "potato chip of the garden." I keep a bowl of these chips next to me when I am catching up on TV time and like to make extra for snacks the next day. Brussels sprouts and other cruciferous vegetables such as broccoli and cauliflower are surprisingly high in protein for vegetables. In addition to fiber, Brussels sprouts deliver a good dose of vitamin C, a powerful antioxidant that fights inflammation.

Feel free to try a different spice blend if you like. You might want to try roasting broccoli or cauliflower for the same health benefits. In fact, you can roast almost any vegetable for a crunchy snack. My philosophy is that when you snack, you might as well eat something healthy.

2 cups Brussels sprouts, trimmed

2 tablespoons olive oil

1½ teaspoons Bayou Cajun Spice Blend (page 235)

1 tablespoon lemon zest

Preheat the oven to 350°F. Line a baking sheet with parchment paper.

Separate the Brussels sprout leaves. They typically yield 5 or 6 leaves per sprout. You want as many leaves as possible.

In a large bowl, combine the olive oil, Bayou Cajun Spice Blend, and lemon zest.

Toss the Brussels sprouts with the olive oil mixture to coat well. Spread the leaves on the lined baking sheet and bake, turning every 5 minutes, until the Brussels sprouts are browned and crispy. Be careful not to burn the chips.

CRISPY AVOCADO CHIPS

Serves: 4
Serving Size: ½ avocado
Calories per serving: 381

No, this isn't a typo. You can make avocado chips that are crispy on the outside and creamy on the inside. I use the Fiesta Spice Blend in this recipe, but you can try any of the spice blends for these "chips."

2 large Hass avocados, pitted, peeled, and sliced into ½-inch wedges

Juice of ½ lime

1 tablespoon Fiesta Spice Blend (page 236)

1 large egg, beaten

¼ cup grated Parmigiano Reggiano cheese

½ teaspoon red pepper flakes

1 cup pumpkin seeds, finely chopped to bread crumb consistency

½ teaspoon lime zest

Olive oil, for drizzling

Preheat the oven to 400°F. Line a baking sheet with parchment paper.

Toss the sliced avocados with the lime juice for flavor and to prevent browning. Add the Fiesta Spice Blend and toss to coat.

Put the beaten egg in a small bowl. In a separate bowl, combine the cheese, red pepper flakes, pumpkin seeds, and lime zest.

Dip the avocado slices in the egg mix and then dredge the slices in the cheese mixture to coat. Arrange them in a single layer on the lined baking sheet and drizzle with olive oil.

Bake for 15 minutes, or until golden.

BARS

CHEF JUDSON'S "PEACH COBBLER" POWER BAR

Yields: 8 bars
Serving size: 1 bar
Calories per serving: 240

What is better than a peach cobbler? Not much as far as I'm concerned. You won't find anything like this bar on grocery store shelves. You will look forward to treating yourself to these irresistible snacks. Wrap them in wax paper, and store them in the refrigerator. They freeze well, too, so you can always have some on hand.

PEACH COBBLER FILLING:

2 cups frozen peaches (thawed, chopped)

2 tablespoons ground flaxseeds

1 teaspoon ground cinnamon

½ teaspoon nutmeg

CRUST:

2 ripe bananas (mashed)

1¼ cup gluten-free oat flour

1¼ cup old-fashioned gluten-free oats

¼ cup pumpkin seeds (chopped)

1 teaspoon cinnamon

2¼ tablespoons maple syrup

1 tablespoon olive oil

Preheat the oven to 350°F.

Peach Cobbler Filling:

Thaw the frozen peaches, and chop them on a cutting board. Make sure to keep all the liquid and juice from the peaches, and add everything to a medium bowl. Add the flaxseeds, ground cinnamon, and nutmeg.

Crust:

Add bananas to a medium bowl, and mash with a potato masher or fork. Combine the flour, oats, pumpkin seeds, cinnamon, maple syrup, and oil. Mix together to form a dough consistency. Reserve 1 cup for the top.

Spray an 8-by-8-inch baking pan with oil, and spread crust evenly on the bottom.

Next add the peach mixture to the top of the crust. Top the peaches with the remaining crust.

Bake for 25 minutes or until golden on top. Cool to solidify, and cut into 8 2-by-4-inch bars.

SOUPS

There is something cozy about having a pot of soup simmering on the stove. From bone broth to corn bisque, this section gives you a range of soups unlike any you have ever tasted. What's great about soup is that you can freeze it in single portions and have a meal ready for you at any time—no muss, no fuss.

BASIC BONE BROTH

Serves: 4
Serving size: 1 cup
Calories per serving: 15

Every four-star restaurant has a big stockpot simmering on a back burner all day long, because freshly made broth has great flavor and endless uses in the kitchen. You can use broth in soups, stews, sauces, and reductions. I like to sip on broth throughout the day. Bone broth is a powerful health tonic that soothes and boosts the immune system.

This recipe calls for beef bones, but broth can be made from beef, lamb, poultry, or fish with vegetables and spices. You can usually get broth-worthy bones from any good butcher or the meat department of your local grocery store, especially if you ask for them ahead of time.

I recommend having a supply of bone broth in your freezer. You can freeze the broth in ice cube trays and store them in a plastic bag once frozen. Freezing bone broth in small portions makes it easy to use it in your everyday cooking.

If you are concerned about leaving the bone broth to simmer on the stovetop largely unattended for 8 to 12 hours, use a large slow cooker set on Low or Medium.

4 pounds beef bones, preferably a mix of marrow bones, oxtail bones, short rib bones, and knuckle bones

2 medium carrots, unpeeled, cut into 2-inch pieces

1 medium leek, cut into 2-inch pieces

1 cup fresh mushrooms (any variety will work)

1 medium yellow onion, quartered

¼ cup chopped fresh parsley

10 garlic cloves, smashed and halved

2 celery stalks, cut into 2-inch pieces

2 bay leaves

1 tablespoon whole black peppercorns

12 cups water

1 tablespoon apple cider vinegar

1 teaspoon fresh lemon juice

Preheat the oven to 450°F.

On a parchment-lined rimmed baking sheet or roasting pan, toss the bones with the carrots, leek, mushrooms, onion, parsley, garlic, celery, bay leaves, peppercorns, vinegar, and lemon juice and roast for 25 minutes.

Stir the ingredients around, then roast for an additional 15 minutes.

Transfer the roasted ingredients to a 6-quart stockpot.

Add 12 cups of water and bring to a boil. Reduce the heat and simmer slowly for 8 to 24 hours, skimming the foam and fat from the top occasionally. The longer you simmer, the more flavorful your broth will be.

When finished, remove from the heat and strain thoroughly, using cheesecloth or a fine-mesh strainer, discarding the solids. Press the ingredients to extract every drop of liquid.

I freeze broth in ice cube trays and transfer the cubes into sealed plastic freezer bags, so that I have small quantities on hand to use in other recipes. I use broth to sauté without using oil.

COCONUT SQUASH SOUP

Serves: 4
Serving size: 1½ cups
Calories per serving: 162

Although this soup is simple to prepare, the blend of flavors is a knockout. Family and friends will think it took you hours to make. I like to have a bowl of it for lunch with a chopped salad on the side.

1 pound butternut squash, peeled and cut into cubes (4 cups)

1 tablespoon olive oil

½ cup chopped onion

1 teaspoon fresh thyme, or ¼ teaspoon dried

⅛ teaspoon dried sage

1 teaspoon honey

1 teaspoon sea salt

1 cup light unsweetened coconut milk

2 cups low-sodium vegetable stock

¼ teaspoon ground turmeric

1¼ teaspoons ground nutmeg

Fresh sage leaves, for garnish (optional)

Preheat the oven to 400°F. Line a baking sheet with parchment paper.

In a large bowl, toss the squash with the olive oil, onion, thyme, sage, honey, and salt. Place on the lined baking sheet and roast for 35 minutes, or until golden.

Transfer the ingredients to a blender and add the coconut milk and vegetable stock. Blend until smooth. If needed, add more stock or coconut milk to thin the soup.

Pour the mixture into a large pot. Add the turmeric and nutmeg and cook for 20 minutes over medium heat, stirring occasionally, to develop flavors. Serve garnished with fresh sage leaves.

CHIPOTLE CHICKEN AND BLACK BEAN SOUP

Serves: 10
Serving size: 2¼ cups
Calories per serving: 380

This Mexican-inspired soup sticks to your ribs and is a complete meal in a bowl. It also freezes well. Garnish with fresh avocado and cilantro after you defrost.

To save time, you can use a rotisserie chicken purchased from the grocery store. Remove the skin and shred the meat with a fork. You can also use left-over cooked chicken breasts for this recipe.

- 1 poblano pepper, diced
- 4 tomatillos, husked, rinsed well, and diced
- 1 cup diced yellow onion
- 12 garlic cloves, minced
- 1 tablespoon olive oil
- 2 pounds boneless, skinless chicken breasts, or 1 rotisserie chicken, skin removed and meat shredded
- 8 cups low-sodium chicken stock
- Juice of 4 limes
- 4 canned chipotle chiles in adobo sauce, minced, sauce reserved
- 1 teaspoon smoked paprika
- 1 (14-ounce) can black beans, drained and rinsed
- ¼ cup finely chopped fresh cilantro
- 2 avocados, pitted, peeled, and diced

Preheat the oven to 400°F. Line a baking sheet with parchment paper.

In a large bowl, toss the poblano pepper, tomatillo, onion, and garlic with the oil. Spread on the lined baking sheet. Roast for 15 to 20 minutes.

If you are using leftover cooked chicken breasts or skinless shredded rotisserie chicken, you can bypass the next step. Cut the leftover chicken breasts into 1-inch cubes.

While your vegetables are roasting, in a saucepan, heat 3 tablespoons of stock over medium-low heat. Add the chicken breasts and sauté until cooked through, about 15 minutes, turning once. Adding stock to the skillet to sauté the chicken is a healthy way to sauté without using oil. Cut the chicken into 1-inch cubes.

Transfer the roasted vegetables to a blender and pulse until smooth. Pour the blended ingredients into a large pot. Add the chicken, stock, lime juice, chipotle peppers and adobo sauce from the can, smoked paprika, black beans, and some of the cilantro. Simmer for 15 minutes. The longer you let this soup simmer, the more pronounced the flavor will be. Add water to taste if the soup seems too strong.

Garnish with the avocado and cilantro.

DINNER

I like to pull out all the stops when it comes to dinner and enjoy preparing an elaborate meal. I'm not saying I like to eat that way every night, but it is fun to treat yourself every now and then. You will see that the main courses I have included in the Phase 1 recipes are quick to prepare—and are just about failproof. The "wow" factor of these recipes will make you glad to be in the kitchen and will delight the family and friends you cook for.

CHINESE SWEET-AND-SPICY CHICKEN KEBABS WITH EASY RELISH

Serves: 4
Serving size: 2 skewers
Calories per serving: 254

If you are making these kebabs for guests, I advise that you to double the recipe. People can't get enough of sweet-and-spicy chicken kebabs, which appear on the cover of this book. When you have moved on to Phase 2, you can serve the skewers over beautiful quinoa with cilantro and red peppers or vegetables.

FOR THE CHICKEN:

1 tablespoon olive oil

¼ teaspoon Chinese five-spice powder

1 tablespoon honey

1 teaspoons sambal oelek (chile paste)

1½ teaspoons Sriracha

1 teaspoon minced garlic

1 tablespoon rice vinegar

1 pound boneless, skinless chicken breasts, cut into 1½-inch cubes or strips

Nonstick cooking spray

FOR THE RELISH:

8 scallions, thinly sliced

1 serrano pepper, sliced

1 tablespoon minced garlic

1 tablespoon minced fresh ginger

1½ tablespoons honey

¼ cup low-sodium soy sauce

1 tablespoon fresh lime juice

1 teaspoon sesame seeds, plus more for garnish

Effortless Thai Fried "Rice" (page 157) or Basic Cauliflower Rice (page 179), for serving

Make the chicken: if you are using wooden skewers, soak them in water for at least 30 minutes.

In a large bowl, combine the olive oil, five-spice powder, honey, sambal oelek, Sriracha, garlic, and vinegar. Reserve 1 tablespoon of the mixture for the finished chicken. Add the chicken cubes or strips to the bowl of marinade, cover, and refrigerate for at least 20 minutes.

Position a rack about 6 inches from the broiler and turn the heat on high. Line a baking sheet with aluminum foil and coat the foil with cooking spray.

Skewer the chicken pieces, place them on the prepared baking sheet, and broil until well browned, 6 to 7 minutes. Flip and broil until the chicken is cooked through, about an additional 4 minutes.

Make the relish: In a medium bowl, combine all the relish ingredients and whisk until fully blended.

Place broiled chicken skewers on a platter and pour the reserved marinade and relish on the chicken. Garnish with additional sesame seeds.

Serve over fried cauliflower rice or simple cauliflower rice.

RUSTIC CHICKEN SAUSAGE STEW

Serves: 6
Serving size: 2 cups
Calories per serving: 384

I can remember eating country food like this satisfying stew at my grand-parents' house. You'll see—the recipe is the peak of comfort food. You can whip up this hardy stew in a little more than an hour. It will fill you up the right way!

1 medium yellow onion, chopped

½ cup chopped red bell pepper

1 cup well-cleaned chopped leeks

1 teaspoon dried thyme

3 vine-ripened tomatoes, chopped

2 tablespoons olive oil, divided

1 pound spicy chicken sausage, sliced into ½-inch-thick coins

1½ tablespoons minced garlic

1 tablespoon fresh lemon juice

3 cups low-sodium beef stock

⅓ cup red wine

2 or 3 bay leaves

2 (14-ounce) cans cannellini beans, drained and rinsed

1 cup low-sodium tomato sauce

3 cups chopped kale

1½ tablespoons Bayou Cajun Spice Blend (page 235)

¼ cup chopped fresh parsley

Preheat the oven to 425°F. Line a baking sheet with parchment paper.

Place the onion, bell pepper, leeks, thyme, and tomatoes on the lined baking sheet and drizzle with 2 teaspoons of the olive oil. Roast for 30 minutes.

In a large Dutch oven or a heavy cooking pot with a lid, heat the remaining olive oil over medium heat. Add the sausage and cook until nicely seared. Add the garlic and stir to incorporate it.

Remove the roasted vegetables from the oven and add to the Dutch oven. Add the lemon juice, stock, wine, and bay leaves and bring to a boil.

Add the beans, tomato sauce, kale, and Creole Spice Blend to the stew. Stir well, cover the pot, and cook over low heat for 30 minutes.

Serve garnished with the parsley.

"ZOODLES" AND CREAMY ROASTED TOMATO SAUCE

Serves: 8
Serving size: 1 cup
Calories per serving: 153

If you find yourself dreaming of pasta, try making pasta from vegetables. Zoodles are made from zucchini. You can make them yourself or buy them prepared at your grocery store. This tomato sauce has many uses. It's luxuriously creamy!

1 pound vine-ripened tomatoes

2 medium yellow onions, chopped

½ cup chopped carrots

6 garlic cloves, chopped

2 medium red bell peppers, cut into spears

2 teaspoons dried oregano

1 to 2 tablespoons olive oil, plus more for serving

⅓ cup red wine

1 tablespoon fresh lemon juice

1 (14-ounce) can low-sodium tomato sauce

¼ cup grated Parmigiano Reggiano cheese

2 tablespoon bottled capers, rinsed

⅓ cup plain nonfat Greek yogurt

1 cup fresh basil leaves, stacked and cut into thin strips, plus more for serving

1 tablespoon finely chopped parsley

1 pound fresh "zoodles" (zucchini noodles)

Preheat the oven at 400°F. Put a large pot of water on to boil for the zoodles.

Line a baking sheet with parchment paper.

Place the tomatoes, onions, carrots, garlic, and bell peppers on the lined baking sheet. Sprinkle with the oregano, drizzle with the olive oil, and roast for 15 to 20 minutes.

Transfer the roasted vegetables to a blender. Add the wine and lemon juice and blend until smooth.

Pour the contents of the blender into a stockpot and add the tomato sauce, cheese, and capers. Simmer for 10 minutes. Add yogurt, basil, and parsley.

Drop the zucchini noodles into the boiling water and cook until al dente. They get soggy quickly, so check for doneness after 3 minutes.

Toss the noodles with the sauce. Garnish with basil and a drizzle of olive oil.

QUICK-AND-EASY JAMAICAN RED SNAPPER ESCOVITCH

Serves: 4
Serving size: 1 fillet
Calories per serving: 201

You can bring island flavors to your kitchen with red snapper *escovitch*. I learned how to make this dish during one of my food excursions to Jamaica. I instantly fell in love with the vinegary sweet heat that "slapped" my taste buds. My spin on this traditional Jamaican fried fish dish retains the peppery, vinegary vegetable sauce, but you will be baking the fish instead of frying it. The Jamaican Me Crazy Spice Blend that you rub into the fillets will give the fish extra kick. You can use commercial jerk seasoning as long as it's low sodium. As they say in Jamaica, "Don't worry, be happy." This delicious recipe will put a smile on your face.

4 red snapper fillets

1½ tablespoons Jamaican Me Crazy Jerk Spice Blend (page 237)

2 tablespoons olive oil, divided

1 white onion, chopped

¼ teaspoon minced garlic

1 cup shredded or matchstick-cut carrots

2 red bell peppers, cut into spears

2 teaspoons fresh thyme

2 allspice berries, cracked

¼ habanero chile, seeded and minced (optional)

¼ cup distilled white vinegar

1 teaspoon honey

Preheat the oven to 400°F.

Place the fish fillets on a baking sheet. Sprinkle the jerk seasoning on each snapper fillet and drizzle with two teaspoons olive oil. Massage the spice blend into the flesh. Set aside.

In a skillet, heat the remaining olive oil over medium-high heat. Add the onion, garlic, carrots, and bell pepper. Cook, stirring, for 1 to 2 minutes. Add the thyme, allspice, habanero, vinegar, honey, and 1 tablespoon water. Cook until the vegetables are softened and the liquid has reduced, about 5 minutes.

Put the fish in the oven and bake for 7 to 10 minutes. Check after 7 minutes. Do not overcook. You want the fish to be moist and tender.

Serve the fish topped with the vegetable mixture.

GOLDEN BBQ CHICKEN

Serves: 8

Serving size: 1 breast

Calories per serving: 260

You can have summer all year long with this oven-baked BBQ chicken! The honey-apricot sauce is divine. Build in marinating time for extra flavor. It is also delicious on fish, shrimp, and pork tenderloin. I like to serve it with roasted seasonal vegetables or over a bed of sautéed collards or gorgeous colored carrots.

FOR THE HONEY-APRICOT BBQ SAUCE:

¾ cup low-sodium tomato sauce

3 tablespoons tomato paste

8 to 10 dried apricots, chopped

2 tablespoons raw honey

½ canned chipotle chile in adobo sauce, plus 1 tablespoon adobo sauce from the can

2 tablespoons Worcestershire sauce

2 tablespoons apple cider vinegar

½ small onion, chopped

2 garlic cloves, finely chopped

¼ cup beer

1 tablespoon smoked paprika

FOR THE CHICKEN:

8 chicken breasts, boneless and skinless

1 tablespoon olive oil

1 tablespoon finely chopped fresh parsley, for garnish

Make the sauce: In a saucepot, add all the sauce ingredients and whisk to combine. Simmer over medium heat for 20 to 30 minutes.

Remove from the heat and carefully transfer the sauce to a blender. Blend until rich and smooth (be careful when blending hot liquids). Let cool for 30 minutes.

Make the chicken: Place chicken parts in a large bowl. Add the olive oil and ¼ cup of the BBQ sauce. Make sure the chicken is fully coated. For ultimate flavor, let the chicken marinate in the refrigerator for 4 to 24 hours.

Preheat the oven to 400°F. Line a baking sheet with aluminum foil.

Place the marinated chicken on the lined baking sheet. Roast for about 30 minutes, until browned and slightly charred on the ends. Finish the chicken with more sauce and sprinkle with the parsley.

SALADS AND SIDES

You can pep up square meals with very little effort. A salad can add some color and lots of flavor and can be anything but bland. Why shouldn't everything on your plate be exceptional? I hope the recipes I have included in this section will inspire you to create your own outstanding sides and salads.

CHARRED MOROCCAN BROCCOLINI

Serves: 2
Serving Size: ¾ cup
Calories per serving: 128

In case you are not familiar with this vegetable, I will introduce you to a new treat. Broccolini looks like baby broccoli or broccoli rabe. It has smaller florets than broccoli and longer, thinner stems. It is sweeter and nuttier than broccoli rabe and broccoli. If you cannot find Broccolini, then broccoli will work just fine in this recipe. I've selected a Moroccan flavor profile with my Moroccan Spice Blend for this dish. You should experiment with other blends. In fact, this is a good basic recipe for broiling all types of vegetables, and you can use just about any of the spice blends to change up this simple side dish. It's a good way to put crunch into your meals and snacks.

4 cups Broccolini, hard ends removed

1 tablespoon olive oil

1½ tablespoons fresh lemon juice

⅛ teaspoon sea salt

2 teaspoons Moroccan Spice Blend (page 241)

Preheat the broiler. Line a baking sheet with parchment paper.

In a large bowl, combine the Broccolini, olive oil, lemon juice, salt, and Moroccan Spice Blend. Stir well to combine.

Spread the spiced Broccolini on the lined baking sheet and broil for 10 minutes, turning two or three times, until the Broccolini florets are crispy and slightly charred.

BASIC CAULIFLOWER RICE

Serves: 4
Serving size: 2 cups
Calories per serving: 268

This is a basic recipe for making cauliflower rice from scratch, which is significantly less expensive than buying a bag of prepared cauliflower. Cooked this way, the "rice" is a simple side dish. You can jazz it up by using different spice blends; adding diced carrots, peppers, and celery for sautéing; or stirring in leftover or steamed vegetables. Cauliflower rice is so much better than starchy, processed rice that you won't miss that simple carbohydrate.

I head cauliflower, separated into florets, stems completely removed

I tablespoon olive oil

¼ cup finely diced yellow onion

2 garlic cloves, finely minced

2 tablespoons finely chopped fresh parsley

Juice of ½ lemon

Working in two batches, pulse half the cauliflower florets in a food processor or blender just until broken down into pieces resembling rice.

In a large skillet, heat the olive oil over medium-high heat. Add the onion and garlic and cook for 3 minutes, then add the cauliflower rice and cook, stirring occasionally, for an additional 5 minutes.

Transfer to a bowl and add the parsley and lemon juice. Stir to incorporate and serve.

SOUTHERN COLLARD GREENS

Serves: 3 to 4
Serving size: ¾ cup
Calories per serving: 172

There was always a place for a bowl of collard greens at my dad's holiday dinners, especially at Thanksgiving. Of course, I was tasked with the glorious job of judging which family member had the best recipe. Let's just say I kept food in my mouth until that topic died down.

Collard greens are a traditional side dish in the South, and Southerners are definitely onto something. Collard greens, along with bok choy, kale, broccoli, Brussels sprouts, cabbage, and turnips, are a member of the cruciferous vegetable family. These veggies are highly nutritious, rich in vitamins A, C, and K, and packed with minerals.

I've dropped the ham hocks from my version of the side dish and replaced them with veggie stock. The greens are delicious enough without the added fat.

I bunch collard greens, thick stems removed

I tablespoon olive oil

I shallot, thinly sliced

I garlic clove, minced

1½ teaspoons red wine vinegar

½ cup vegetable stock

Roll the collard leaves together like a tight cigar and cut them crosswise into thin strips. This is called chiffonade.

In a skillet, heat the olive oil over medium-high heat. Add the shallot and garlic and cook for 1 minute.

Add the collard greens, vinegar, and vegetable stock and cook until the collards are bright green and tender, about 4 minutes.

GRILLED PEACH AND KALE SALAD

Serves: 4
Serving Size: ⅔ cup
Calories per serving: 111

The summer brings about family, fun, and of course your relatives' "signature" must-have side dishes. Create a standout crowd-pleaser and try this nontraditional vegetarian side dish that demands attention because of its striking colors and bold flavors. The peaches are grilled until caramelized, sweet, and juicy. If you can't grill them outside, use a grill pan or broiler. Paired with kale greens, unsalted roasted sunflower seeds for crunch, dried cranberries, and balsamic vinegar, this salad is a superstar.

2 to 3 bunches kale, thick stems
  removed

2 ripe peaches, pitted and cut into
  wedges

½ teaspoon olive oil

2 tablespoons dried cranberries

2 tablespoons roasted unsalted
  sunflower seeds

¼ cup balsamic vinegar

Stack the kale leaves on top of one another and roll them up like a cigar. Cut them crosswise into thin strips. This method of preparation is called chiffonade. Place the kale strips in a bowl and set aside.

In a medium bowl, toss the peach wedges with the olive oil until they are fully coated. Cover and refrigerate for about 15 minutes.

Heat a charcoal or gas grill to 400°F.

Cook the peaches until charred, soft, and caramelized. Remove from the grill and set aside in a heat-resistant bowl.

Add the cranberries and sunflower seeds to the bowl with the kale. Top with the grilled peaches. Serve with the balsamic vinegar on the side for drizzling.

DESSERTS

I never said you had to give up dessert! That wouldn't be realistic, especially if you have a sweet tooth. I have spent a lot of time and effort coming up with indulgent desserts that do not rely on processed sugar and heavy cream. Keep some sorbets and "ice cream," recipes for which you will find in this section, in the freezer to ensure you can satisfy a sweet craving without falling off the wagon. And don't forget the truffles!

DRUNKEN ALMONDS

Serves: 8
Serving size: 23 almonds
Calories per serving: 214

The mellow sweetness of these almonds puts them in the dessert category for me. They go well with a bowl of fresh berries or slices of pineapple.

3 tablespoons pure maple syrup

3 tablespoons bourbon

½ teaspoon ground cardamom

2 cups raw unsalted almonds

Preheat the oven to 325°F. Line a baking sheet with parchment paper.

In a medium saucepan, combine the maple syrup, bourbon, cardamom, and ⅓ cup water. Bring to a boil. Reduce the heat to medium and simmer for 15 minutes.

Take the pan off the heat, add the almonds, and let them sit in the syrup for 35 minutes.

Transfer the almonds to the lined baking sheet. Roast for 10 to 15 minutes, or until the almonds are dry and golden. You can store these nuts in an airtight container for nine months to a year in the pantry, 1 year in the refrigerator, and up to two years in the freezer.

SUMMER DAY SORBET

Serves: 4
Serving size: ½ cup
Calories per serving: 69

Making sorbet in your kitchen is a snap. You should keep a container of sorbet in your freezer in case your sweet tooth acts up. I love the combination of strawberries and basil in this recipe, but there are endless possibilities. Check the fruit and spice compatibility chart (see page 250) to create your signature sorbet.

1 pound hulled fresh or frozen
    strawberries

¼ cup finely chopped fresh basil leaves

2 tablespoons honey

1½ cups water

Combine all the ingredients and 1½ cups water in a blender and pulse until smooth.

Transfer to a metal bowl or other container, cover with a lid or plastic wrap, and freeze. Or freeze the mixture in an ice cream machine according to the manufacturer's instructions.

TROPICAL SORBET

Serves: 4
Serving size: ½ cup
Calories per serving: 73

This refreshing sorbet is very tropical. If you keep it in the freezer, you will be able satisfy and indulge your taste buds anytime without going off track.

I mango, pitted, peeled, cut into cubes, and frozen

I cup pineapple, cubed and frozen

I teaspoon lime zest

I tablespoon fresh lime juice

⅛ teaspoon cayenne pepper

½ cup ice cubes

I cup water

Combine all the ingredients in a blender and blend until smooth. Transfer to a metal bowl, cover with plastic wrap, and freeze to the desired consistency, at least 2 hours.

BUTTERY MACADAMIA NUT "ICE CREAM"

Serves: 4
Serving size: ½ cup
Calories per serving: 147

No cream or sugar is needed in this recipe. Instead, bananas are used to make the "ice cream." The buttery macadamia nuts add the crunch and contribute to the rich flavor. You can serve this "ice cream" frozen or semifreddo—"half cold"—as the Italians do.

3 ripe bananas, peeled, sliced, and frozen

I tablespoon pure vanilla extract

3 tablespoons unsweetened almond milk

¼ cup finely chopped macadamia nuts

Place the bananas, vanilla, and almond milk in a food processor and process until smooth and creamy.

Scoop into a chilled bowl and fold in the macadamia nuts.

Serve immediately as soft serve, or transfer to the freezer until hardened to the desired consistency, about 2 hours.

HAZELNUT DARK CHOCOLATE TRUFFLES

Yields: 8
Serving size: 2 truffles
Calories per serving: 96

All I can say is "yum!" The Spice Diet takes care of chocoholics and sweet lovers.

I cup unsweetened dark cocoa powder

I teaspoon orange zest

¼ cup fresh orange juice

I teaspoon dark rum

3 tablespoons pure maple syrup

⅓ cup finely chopped toasted hazelnuts

Combine the cocoa powder and orange zest in a small bowl. Make a well in the center and pour in the orange juice, rum, and maple syrup. Stir until the ingredients are completely blended. Chill the chocolate mixture for at least 30 minutes.

Line a baking sheet with parchment paper. Remove the chocolate mixture from the refrigerator, roll into small balls about ½ inch across, and coat with the crushed hazelnuts. Serve chilled.

Read on if you want to see how you will be eating in Phase 2. The foods and menus are not radically different from Phase 1, except you can eat more calories and are able to add some starchy carbs. I have included a few exotic recipes in Phase 2 that are so spectacular you won't believe the finished product came out of your kitchen. You will not feel deprived when you eat the Spice Diet way.

10

POWERHOUSE FLAVOR RECIPES FOR PHASE 2

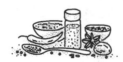

Congratulations! If you are ready to move on to Phase 2, you must be close to reaching your goals. Take a picture of yourself for your vision board. Look over your notes on conquering your addictions and eliminating junk food from your daily menus. You have been following the Spice Diet way of eating for at least a month. Your taste buds must be thanking you. You must be getting accustomed to eating healthy, fresh food. A craving might pop up now and then—they never really disappear completely—but now you have plenty of ways to satisfy your cravings with smoothies, snacks, and desserts that feel very indulgent.

I hope you are ready for more adventures in knockout flavor! I am crazy about the foods of all nations and have included flavor profiles from many different cultures in my Phase 2 recipes. Having tried the Phase 1 recipes, you have embraced the big, bold flavors I love and have enjoyed the exotic and unconventional flavor combinations that comprise my signature style of cooking.

In Phase 2, your daily calorie count is bumped up. You can now add some starchy carbs to your diet, including whole wheat pasta, brown rice, quinoa, sweet potatoes, and corn, to name a few welcome additions. These carbs can add another dimension to your diet, although you do have to stay mindful of portion control. If you are eating any grain or starch as a main course keep it to 1 cup for your serving. As a side dish, your portion should be ½ cup.

From an Almond "PB&J" Protein Smoothie to Candied Chickpeas, from Veggie Taquitos to South-of-the-Border Grilled Corn Soup, from Steve Harvey's Favorite Lobster Mac and Cheese to Decadent Peanut Butter Cup "Ice Cream," my Phase 2 recipes will continue to expand your palate with "food-gasmic" flavor.

Phase 2 is the way you should eat for the rest of your life. If you find yourself indulging too often and your weight starts to creep up, return to Phase 1—and of course keep using any of those recipes that you like during Phase 2! My rule of thumb is, if you gain five pounds or more, revisit the Phase 1 meal plans. You have put in a lot of effort to get where you are, and you don't want those old eating habits to take a wrecking ball to your resolve. It's a comfort to know that you can reset your diet anytime you want without having to give up delicious food.

You have probably developed a sense of how to put spices together with healthy ingredients. If you didn't think of yourself as a cook before, I hope you are gaining confidence in the kitchen. I want you to enjoy making food that surpasses what you used to eat. Have fun with the Phase 2 recipes. Feel free to modify them to suit your tastes. The seventy-two Powerhouse Flavor Recipes in this book, plus the twenty-five spice blends that I will introduce to you in chapter 11, are a good foundation for preparing food that is as healthy as it is delicious.

PHASE 2 RECIPES

Breakfast

Savory Oatmeal Bowl (page 188)
"Granola" Oatmeal (page 189)
Lemon-Blueberry Pancakes with Sweet-and-Spicy Syrup (page 189)
Banana-Citrus Yogurt (page 191)

Green Drinks, Juices, and Smoothies

Almond "PB&J" Protein Smoothie (page 192)
Big Red Juice (page 192)

Desserts

Earl Grey–Infused Lemon Granita (page 216)

Chocolate Banana Bites (page 217)

Guiltless Lemon-Blueberry Cake Milk Shake (page 217)

Grandma's Carrot Cake Oatmeal Cookies (page 218)

Decadent Chocolate Peanut Butter Cup "Ice Cream" (page 219)

BREAKFAST

SAVORY OATMEAL BOWL

Serves: 1

Serving size: ½ cup

Calories per serving: 275

When thinking about dressing up oatmeal, most of us go to sweet flavors. This recipe goes against that impulse by adding mushrooms, goat cheese, red pepper flakes for heat, and a bit of honey for sweetness. Savory oatmeal is so delicious, you will want to eat it any time of day!

½ teaspoon honey

2 tablespoons skim milk

½ cup old-fashioned rolled oats

1 teaspoon olive oil

½ cup sliced cremini mushrooms

⅛ teaspoon chopped fresh thyme

⅛ teaspoon red pepper flakes

1½ tablespoons crumbled goat cheese

In a medium saucepan, combine the honey, milk, and ¾ cup water and bring to a boil over medium heat. Stir in the oats. Reduce the heat to medium and simmer, stirring occasionally, for 5 minutes.

Heat the olive oil in a skillet over medium-high heat. Add the mushrooms, thyme, and red pepper flakes and cook, stirring occasionally to prevent burning, until golden and crispy, about 5 minutes.

Top the creamy oatmeal with the mushrooms and crumbled goat cheese.

"GRANOLA" OATMEAL

Serves: 2
Serving size: 1½ cups
Calories per serving: 328

This recipe has all the flavor of granola, but you eat it hot. The oats are soft rather than crispy, but the nuts and dried fruits give the oatmeal great texture. Make sure you buy a supply of nuts and dried fruits, because "Granola" Oatmeal could become your go-to breakfast.

2 cups unsweetened almond milk

1 cup quick-cooking oats or instant oatmeal

1 teaspoon pure vanilla extract

1½ tablespoons pure maple syrup

1 tablespoon finely chopped pecans

1 tablespoon finely chopped cashews

1½ teaspoons raisins

1½ teaspoons unsweetened dried cranberries

1½ teaspoons unsweetened dried cherries

¼ teaspoon ground cinnamon

Bring the almond milk to a boil in a medium pot.

Stir in the oats, vanilla, and maple syrup. Cook for 3 minutes.

Reduce the heat to mediium and add the nuts, dried fruit, and cinnamon. Simmer for 5 minutes, stirring occasionally. Put half the oatmeal in a bowl and enjoy. Save the rest for another day.

LEMON-BLUEBERRY PANCAKES WITH SWEET-AND-SPICY SYRUP

Serves: 4
Serving size: 3 (3-inch) pancakes plus 1 tablespoon syrup
Calories per serving: 394

Now that you are at Phase 2, you can have a bit more flour in your diet, though not white flour. My take on blueberry pancakes will be a great weekend treat. I have added fresh lemon zest, because it lifts the flavor. Many of the nutrients and much of the flavor in a lemon are in the peel.

To speed up the pancake-making process, you can purchase gluten-free pancake mix, which contains no white or wheat flour. If you don't want the added sugar from the honey in the syrup, you can top your pancakes with nonfat yogurt or fresh fruit. Always remember you can make your food your own and modify recipes to suit your taste. If you are not a fan of blueberries, then swap them out for your favorite fruit, such as strawberries or apples dusted with cinnamon.

FOR THE PANCAKES:

1⅓ cups almond flour

1 tablespoon baking powder

½ teaspoon sea salt

1 large egg

¾ cup unsweetened almond milk

1 tablespoon sugar

2 tablespoons olive oil

2 teaspoons lemon zest

1 teaspoon fresh lemon juice

½ cup fresh blueberries

Nonstick cooking spray

FOR THE SWEET-AND-SPICY SYRUP:

1 cup raw honey

½ teaspoon grated fresh ginger

Make the pancakes: Combine the flour, baking powder, and salt. In another bowl, beat the egg until frothy. Mix in the almond milk, sugar, olive oil, lemon zest, and lemon juice until the ingredients are blended. Mix in the combined dry ingredients until they are completely incorporated.

Gently stir in the blueberries.

Heat a griddle over medium high heat. Spray the griddle with nonstick cooking spray. For each pancake, pour 3 to 4 tablespoons of batter onto the griddle and cook until puffed and dry around the edges. Flip and cook the other side until golden brown.

Make the syrup: In a saucepot, combine the honey, grated ginger, and 1 tablespoon water and whisk thoroughly. Cook for 10 minutes over low heat until slightly warm.

Drizzle the syrup over hot and ready-to-go pancakes.

BANANA-CITRUS YOGURT

Serves: 2
Serving size: 1 cup
Calories per serving: 312

This yogurt treat has a lot going on—the tartness of grapefruit, the creaminess of banana, the lift of mint, and the crunch of macadamia nuts provide layered flavor and texture.

I medium pink grapefruit

I teaspoon pure vanilla extract

I tablespoon honey

I tablespoon chopped fresh mint

I banana, sliced

2 cups plain nonfat Greek yogurt

1½ tablespoons chopped macadamia nuts

Slice off the skin and white pith from the grapefruit. Cut the segments from their surrounding membranes to release the grapefruit segments into a medium bowl.

Add the vanilla, honey, banana, and mint. Toss gently.

Spoon the fruit mixture over the yogurt and top with the macadamia nuts.

GREEN DRINKS, JUICES, AND SMOOTHIES

If you have smoothie left over, I don't recommend refrigerating what remains, because the ingredients of the smoothie will separate and the drink loses its thickness and becomes more liquid. Instead, put the leftover smoothie in an airtight container and freeze it. You can thaw the smoothie overnight and simply reblend with additional fruit, if you would like, and have no prep time for your morning meal.

ALMOND "PB&J" PROTEIN SMOOTHIE

Serves: 2
Serving size: 1½ cups
Calories per serving: 367

Talk about comfort food! A sip of this smoothie will be a nostalgic reminder of your childhood—those peanut butter and jelly sandwich days. Given that peanuts are higher in fat than most nut options, we are substituting with almonds. While the flavor profile of these nuts is quite different, this smoothie certainly satisfies that sweet and savory tooth.

¼ cup natural unsweetened almond butter

¼ cup frozen raspberries

¼ cup frozen blueberries

⅔ cup frozen strawberries

1 cup unsweetened almond milk

1 banana

1 tablespoon vanilla protein powder

Combine all the ingredients in a blender and blend until well mixed. Pour into glasses and share.

BIG RED JUICE

Serves: 2
Serving size: 1 cup
Calories per serving: 80

Big Red Juice is sweet and refreshing, with a little bite from the ginger. And the color is extraordinary!

2 cups cubed seeded watermelon

1 beet, quartered

1 carrot

1 (1-inch) piece fresh ginger

Run all the ingredients through a juicer.

If you do not have a juicer, combine all the ingredients with ¼ cup water in a blender and blend until smooth. Strain the mixture through a fine-mesh strainer or a colander lined with cheesecloth to get the pure juice, and discard the pulp.

THE KALE-LEIDOSCOPE GREEN DRINK

Serves: 2
Serving size: 1 cup
Calories per serving: 94

My Kale-leidoscope Green Drink is nutrition-packed. The green apple adds sweetness, the lemon juice contributes just the right amount of tartness, and the coconut water brings another level of flavor to the drink. This green drink is one of the healthiest snacks you can find.

2 celery stalks

½ cucumber

I green apple

I cup tightly packed chopped kale leaves

I sprig parsley

Juice of ½ lemon

¼ cup unsweetened coconut water

Combine all the ingredients in a blender and blend until smooth. Pour into glasses and enjoy!

ALOHA SODA

Serves: 2 or 3
Serving size: 1½ cups
Calories per serving: 65

I was one of those people who was addicted to soda! It's as if I had to have one every time I ate. I felt like the "free refill" concept for those sugary drinks was designed especially for me! So it's only fair that I share my secret soda alternative with you. The natural sweetness of the fresh fruit offers a much better taste than the canned stuff. Say good-bye to the refined sugar overload for good!

1½ cups fresh or frozen ripe pineapple

Juice of 1 lime

1 tablespoon honey, plus more to taste

3 cups sparkling water

In a blender, combine the pineapple, lime juice, honey, and ⅓ cup water and blend until smooth. Pour the pineapple-lime mixture into a pitcher, add the sparkling water, and stir with a spoon.

For additional sweetness, add more honey, but taste as you go so you don't overdo it. Pour over ice cubes and get ready to be refreshed.

LUNCH

VEGGIE TAQUITOS

Serves: 4
Serving size: 2 taquitos
Calories per serving: 294

Who doesn't love the crispy wonderfulness that taquitos have to offer? Although these cool finger foods are traditionally deep-fried, baking cuts down on your fat intake. Keep in mind that by using corn tortillas you bypass the flour and added fat and salt of flour tortillas. They're made with white maize, a type of corn that is richer in protein and much more nutritious.

2 cups chopped fresh cremini mushrooms

⅓ cup chopped Spanish onion

2 tablespoons chopped fresh poblano pepper

¾ cup thin red bell pepper strips

4 teaspoons olive oil (divided)

8 6-inch corn tortillas

1¼ cups canned black beans, drained and rinsed

2 cups shredded kale

¼ cup shredded Monterey Jack cheese

3 tablespoons Mexican hot sauce

2 tablespoons light sour cream, for garnish (optional)

2 tablespoons thinly sliced scallion

Preheat the oven to 425°F. Line a baking sheet with parchment paper.

Spread the mushrooms, onion, and peppers and coat with 1 teaspoon of oil. Roast for 20 to 25 minutes or until caramelized and tender.

Fill each tortilla with about ⅓ cup of filling, layering black beans, veggies, shredded kale, and cheese. Remember, a little cheese goes a long way so do not overdo it!! Roll up the tortilla as tightly as possible and stick toothpicks in the middle to hold it together.

Place the taquitos seam side down on a parchment-lined baking sheet. Make sure not to place them too closely together. Brush each with the remaining 3 teaspoons of oil.

Bake for 10 to 15 minutes or until golden and crispy. Garnish with a drizzle of your favorite Mexican hot sauce, light sour cream, and scallions.

THE ULTIMATE TUNA SALAD

Serves: 4 to 6
Serving size: 1 cup
Calories per serving: 257

The Ultimate Tuna Salad is extremely rich—even without the mayonnaise. The herbs and spices make this unlike any tuna salad you have ever tasted. It's a party in your mouth!

3 (5-ounce) cans albacore tuna in water, drained

½ English cucumber, diced

1 teaspoon capers, drained

2 avocados, pitted, peeled, and cut into ½-inch cubes

1 small red onion, thinly sliced into half-moons

2 tablespoons finely chopped fresh parsley

½ teaspoon finely chopped fresh dill

2 tablespoons finely chopped fresh cilantro

¾ cup sliced cherry tomatoes

2 teaspoons Bayou Cajun Spice Blend (page 235)

2 tablespoons fresh lemon juice

2 tablespoons olive oil

In a large serving bowl, combine the tuna, cucumber, capers, avocados, onion, fresh herbs, tomatoes, and Cajun Spice Blend.

Add the lemon juice and olive oil and toss the salad.

CHICKEN CAESAR SALAD—HOLD THE ANCHOVIES

Serves: 5
Serving size: 1½ cups salad plus 1 to 2 tablespoons dressing
Calories per serving: 216

In the interest of time, this recipe calls for using a precooked rotisserie chicken. When you select a rotisserie chicken, make certain you buy one that has no salt added. Remember to remove all the skin and fat. I have kept the cheese to a minimum, because a little goes a long way when a recipe has so many ingredients that contribute to the flavor. My twist on a traditional Caesar salad dressing is to use yogurt for creaminess. Dijon mustard and Worcestershire sauce are my secret weapons in this healthier version of dressing. I leave the anchovies out of the traditional Caesar salad dressing, because they are so salty.

FOR THE SALAD:

1½ cups shredded skinless rotisserie chicken

1 small red onion, sliced into half-moons

2 hard-boiled eggs, chopped

½ cup cherry tomatoes, halved

FOR THE DRESSING:

⅓ cup plain nonfat Greek yogurt

2 garlic cloves, minced

2 teaspoons Worcestershire sauce

2 tablespoons fresh lemon juice

1½ teaspoons Dijon mustard

½ teaspoon freshly ground black pepper

2 tablespoons olive oil

2½ tablespoons grated Parmigiano Reggiano cheese

2 heads romaine lettuce, cut into 1½-inch pieces, for serving

Make the salad: in a large bowl, mix together the shredded chicken, onion, eggs, and tomatoes and set aside.

Make the dressing: in a small bowl, combine the yogurt, garlic, Worcestershire, lemon juice, mustard, and pepper. Whisk to combine fully.

While whisking, drizzle in the olive oil. Add the cheese and whisk to combine.

Toss the salad with ¼ cup of the dressing.

Serve over the romaine lettuce.

Save the remaining dressing for a quick and easy salad. It will keep in the refrigerator for two weeks.

SALMON QUINOA BOWL

Serves: 4
Serving size: 4 to 5 ounces salmon plus 1 cup quinoa
Calories per serving: 517

Now that you have reintroduced grains to your diet, you will enjoy this tasty use of the superfood quinoa. The recipe is quick and easy to prepare and packs a serious flavor punch.

Remember that you can always swap out your proteins. For this recipe, I chose a 4-ounce piece of salmon, but this quinoa bowl works great with grilled chicken or lamb.

4 (4- to 5-ounce) pieces skinless salmon

2 tablespoons extra-virgin olive oil, divided

1/8 teaspoon freshly ground black pepper

¼ cup fresh lemon juice

1 tablespoon red wine vinegar

¼ cup finely chopped fresh dill

¼ cup finely chopped fresh mint

2 tablespoons finely chopped fresh oregano

1 cup quinoa

2 cups water

1½ cups halved cherry tomatoes

1 cup assorted pitted olives, such as Kalamata and Gaeta, halved

⅓ cup chopped scallions

1 small red onion, thinly sliced into half-moons

3 cups sliced English cucumbers

⅓ cup crumbled feta cheese

2 tablespoons finely chopped fresh parsley for garnish

Preheat the oven to 425°F. Line a baking sheet with parchment paper.

Lay out the salmon pieces on the lined baking sheet. Brush the fillets with 1 teaspoon of the olive oil and season with pepper. Roast for 10 minutes.

In a large bowl, combine the lemon juice, vinegar, herbs, and remaining olive oil. Whisk until emulsified. Let the dressing sit at room temperature to allow the flavors to meld.

Rinse the quinoa in a strainer until the water runs clear. Combine the quinoa and 2 cups of water in a saucepan and bring to a boil. Reduce the heat to low, cover, and cook until the water has been absorbed, about 15 minutes. The quinoa should be tender.

Transfer the quinoa to a bowl and fluff it with a fork. Add the tomatoes, olives, scallions, red onion, and cucumbers and toss with the dressing. Top with the feta and parsley.

Serve chilled or warm with salmon.

SNACKS AND APPETIZERS

CARAMELIZED SHALLOTS AND SPINACH DIP

Serves: 4 to 6
Serving size: 3 ounces, which is very generous
Calories per serving: 172

My flavorful version makes everyday dips seem bland in comparison. You can serve the dip at room temperature or nuke it briefly to warm it up. I guarantee you will not have any leftovers. If by some miracle there are, store the remaining dip in a covered container in the refrigerator. Use raw or crispy roasted vegetables to scoop up the dip. I like roasted cauliflower or fresh veggies with this dip. Also try baking your own root vegetable chips like beets and sweet potatoes.

I tablespoon plus I teaspoon
   olive oil

4 or 5 shallots, thinly sliced

2 cups plain nonfat Greek yogurt

⅓ cup reduced-fat cream cheese, at
   room temperature

2 tablespoons snipped fresh chives

I teaspoon minced garlic

3 cups tightly packed baby spinach

I tablespoon white wine

⅛ teaspoon freshly ground black
   pepper

In a large skillet, heat 1 teaspoon of the olive oil over medium heat. Add the shallots and cook for 8 to 10 minutes, or until caramelized, stirring occasionally to prevent burning. Set aside.

In a medium bowl, stir together the yogurt, cream cheese, and chives. Fold in the caramelized shallots.

In the same skillet in which the onions were cooked, heat 1 tablespoon of olive oil. Add the garlic and spinach and cook for 2 minutes. Add the wine and scrape the bottom of the pan to release any browned bits. Add the cooked spinach and any liquid from the skillet to the yogurt mixture and stir to combine fully.

Serve with roasted cauliflower or fresh veggies.

CRISPY CAULIFLOWER BITES

Serves: 2 to 4
Serving size: ½ cup
Calories per serving: 175

Cauliflower Bites are golden nuggets of flavor, and they look great on a plate as a side. I suggest you make extra, because they are very satisfying to snack on.

½ cup oat flour or almond flour

2 tablespoons finely chopped fresh chives

1½ tablespoons finely chopped fresh dill

¼ cup red wine vinegar

2 tablespoons olive oil, divided

1 large head cauliflower, cut into small florets

Preheat the oven to 425°F. Line a baking sheet with parchment paper.

In a zip-top bag, combine the oat flour, chives, and dill.

Put the vinegar and 1 tablespoon of the olive oil in a large bowl and whisk until combined. Add the cauliflower and toss to coat. To intensify the flavor, marinate for 30 minutes to 1 hour.

Transfer the cauliflower florets to the zip-top bag and shake to coat. Place the florets on the lined baking sheet. Drizzle the cauliflower with the remaining olive oil.

Bake for 15 minutes, turn the florets, and bake for another 15 minutes. The cauliflower bites are done when they are crispy and golden in color.

CANDIED CHICKPEAS

Serves: 3
Serving size: ½ cup
Calories per serving: 260

This recipe converts humble chickpeas into a crispy, tart, and sweet treat. You might want to consider doubling the recipe. You'll be happy to have plenty of this delicious snack on hand.

1 (15-ounce) can chickpeas, drained and rinsed

½ cup balsamic vinegar

2 tablespoons olive oil

1 tablespoon pure maple syrup

¼ teaspoon freshly ground black pepper

Combine the chickpeas and vinegar in a large bowl. Cover and marinate the chickpeas in the refrigerator for 1 to 2 hours.

Preheat the oven to 375°F. Line a rimmed baking sheet with parchment paper.

Drain the marinated chickpeas and return to the bowl. Add the olive oil, maple syrup, and pepper and toss.

Place the chickpeas on the lined baking sheet. Bake for 25 minutes, or until golden.

QUICK-PICKLED GREEN BEANS

Yield: 2 pints
Serving size: 1 cup
Calories per serving: 73

These used to be called dilly beans, because of the pickling process, which uses dill for flavor. Needless to say, I've amped up the flavor with coriander seeds, red pepper flakes, and ginger. How you flavor your quick-pickled vegetables is all up to you! This is a perfect way to incorporate spices like mustard seed, coriander, peppercorns, and red pepper flakes as well as fresh herbs like dill, rosemary, thyme, and garlic.

Quick pickling involves pickling vegetables in vinegar, water, and salt and storing them in the refrigerator in a covered jar. They only require a few days in the brine before they can be enjoyed, and you don't have to can them.

You get to choose how sour you want them to be. The longer they sit in the brine, the more flavorful they become. To get the best pickled vegetables, start with the freshest vegetables you can find.

I put pickled vegetables in salads and wraps, use them as a side, and snack on them. There is always a jar of something pickling in my fridge.

2 sprigs fresh dill

2 sprigs fresh thyme

1 to 2 teaspoons whole black peppercorns

1 to 2 teaspoons coriander seeds

1 teaspoon red pepper flakes, or to taste

1 teaspoon chopped fresh ginger

2 garlic cloves, sliced

1 pound fresh green beans

1 cup rice vinegar or apple cider vinegar

2 teaspoons sea salt

1½ teaspoons agave nectar

1 cup water

Equipment needed: 2 pint-size, large-mouth mason Jars

Divide the herb sprigs, peppercorns, coriander, red pepper flakes, ginger, and garlic between two sterilized widemouthed mason jars.

Stand the green beans upright in the jars. Make sure there is ½ inch clearance or space from the rim of the jar to the top of the beans.

In a small saucepan, combine the vinegar, sea salt, agave, and 1 cup of water and bring to a boil over high heat, stirring continuously to dissolve the salt. Pour the brine over the beans while hot, filling each jar within ½ inch of the top.

Gently tap the jars against the counter to remove all air bubbles. Place the lids on the jars and screw them on until tight. Store the beans in the refrigerator for 2 to 3 days to pickle.

BARS

CHEF JUDSON'S CITRUS PROTEIN BAR

Yields: 8 bars
Serving size: 1 bar
Calories per serving: 160

My health bars surpass any protein bars you can find in flavor and nutrition. I use only natural sources of sweetness. Wrap them in wax paper, and store them in the refrigerator. Citrus Protein Bars freeze well, too, so make a big batch!

¼ cup quinoa, uncooked

¼ cup macadamia nuts

¼ cup unsweetened coconut flakes, chopped

⅓ cup chickpeas, drained and rinsed

⅓ cup dried pineapple, finely chopped

I scoop vanilla protein powder (use your favorite brand)

I tablespoon lime zest

I tablespoon lime juice

⅓ cup pure honey

I tablespoon coconut oil

I egg white

Preheat the oven to 350°F.

On a lined cooking sheet, add the quinoa and macadamia nuts. Toast for 5–8 minutes or until golden. Add the coconut to the sheet tray, and toast for an additional 2 minutes.

Add the chickpeas to a bowl, and mash them with a fork.

Add the toasted quinoa mixture, dried pineapple, protein powder, lime zest, and lime juice to the bowl. Mix evenly.

Add the honey and oil, and mix well. Add the egg white.

Press the mix into an 8-by-8 lined and oiled baking dish.

Reduce the temperature to 300-degrees, and bake for 35–40 minutes or until golden. Cool and cut into 8 2-by-4-inch bars.

SOUPS

SOUTH-OF-THE-BORDER GRILLED CORN BISQUE

Serves: 4
Serving size: 1½ cups
Calories per serving: 161

This decadent dish is a play on the popular Mexican street food *elotes*, grilled corn with lime and chili powder. It highlights the sweet flavor of locally grown grilled yellow corn in tandem with the spice of hot sauce. Most bisques are laden with heavy cream and butter, but this recipe transforms the bisque to lighter fare by using roasted cauliflower, light coconut milk, and vegetable stock, to add richness to the soup.

Topped with corn kernels, smoked paprika, and cilantro, this soup is simply divine.

6 ears fresh yellow corn, husked

½ medium Vidalia onion, quartered

½ poblano pepper, quartered

½ cup cauliflower florets

3 sprigs fresh thyme

½ teaspoon olive oil

½ cup light unsweetened coconut milk

3 cups low-sodium vegetable stock

2 tablespoons hot sauce or to taste

½ teaspoon chili powder

½ teaspoon smoked paprika

½ teaspoon lime zest

1 teaspoon finely chopped fresh cilantro

Preheat the oven to 400°F. Line a baking sheet with parchment paper.

Put the corn, onion, poblano, cauliflower, and thyme on the lined baking sheet. Drizzle the olive oil over the veggies and roast for 20 to 25 minutes, or until caramelized.

Cut the corn from the cobs into a bowl.

In a blender, combine the roasted veggies, corn kernels, coconut milk, veggie stock, and hot sauce. Blend until smooth and creamy. Transfer the corn bisque to a stockpot and simmer over medium heat for 15 to 20 minutes to allow the flavors to meld.

Serve warm or cold, topped with the chili powder, smoked paprika, lime zest, and cilantro.

THAI SHRIMP RED CURRY SOUP

Serves: 4
Serving size: 2 cups
Calories per serving: 273

This traditional Thai soup is a meal in itself. The ingredients create a harmonious balance between spicy and sweet, which is typical of Thai food and why I enjoy the cuisine so much. This red curry soup is simple to prepare and delivers "orgasmic" flavor.

5 or 6 large carrots, coarsely chopped

1 medium white onion, finely chopped

2 tablespoons olive oil, divided

1 garlic clove, minced

1 tablespoon red curry paste (you can add ½ tablespoon more if you like your food spicy)

1 tablespoon fresh lime juice

1 tablespoon minced fresh ginger

4 cups low-sodium chicken stock

1 teaspoon honey

1 tablespoon finely chopped fresh basil

1 cup light unsweetened coconut milk

1 pound extra-jumbo (16–20 count) shrimp, peeled and deveined

2 scallions, cut into thick strips

2 tablespoons fresh cilantro leaves

Preheat the oven to 400°F. Line a baking sheet with parchment paper.

Put the carrots and onion on the lined baking sheet and toss with 1 tablespoon of the olive oil to coat. Roast for 25 minutes, or until the vegetables are caramelized and tender.

In a large saucepan, heat the remaining 1 tablespoon of olive oil. Add the garlic, red curry paste, lime juice, and ginger and cook for 2 to 3 minutes. Add the chicken stock, honey, basil, and coconut milk and bring to a boil. Reduce the heat to maintain a simmer and cook for 4 minutes. Carefully transfer the coconut milk mixture and the roasted carrots and onion to a blender. Blend until smooth and creamy, about 1 minute. Be careful when blending hot liquids.

Return the blended soup to the saucepot, add the shrimp, and simmer 10 to 15 minutes to bring the flavors together. If the soup is too spicy or thick, you can add more coconut milk or stock.

Ladle the soup into bowls and garnish with the scallions and cilantro.

ONE-POT-WONDER SUPREME SEAFOOD STEW

Serves: 4 to 6
Serving size: 2 cups
Calories per serving: 256

Don't be intimidated by the number of ingredients in this dish—the long list is evidence that you are in for a flavor explosion. This super-simple recipe is one of my favorite one-pot wonders! Typically, one-pot wonders require a slew of ingredients, but the time-saver here is that you throw all your ingredients in the pot or slow cooker and let the stew simmer away.

If the cost of seafood is too expensive or if you are allergic to shellfish, swap it out for chicken and savory turkey sausage. If you are a vegetarian, this recipe works amazingly with white beans as well.

My favorite way to cook this dish is using a slow cooker. If you don't own one, a large stockpot works just as well. We will use a stockpot for this recipe because not everyone owns a slow cooker.

2 tablespoons olive oil

6 garlic cloves, minced

¼ teaspoon red pepper flakes

1 leek, cleaned well and chopped

1 small fennel bulb, chopped

1 teaspoon finely chopped fresh thyme

1 cup halved cherry tomatoes

2 bay leaves

3 cups low-sodium chicken stock

1 cup bottled clam juice

2 tablespoons fresh lemon juice

2 tablespoons tomato paste

½ cup white wine

½ pound medium shrimp, peeled and deveined

½ pound white-fleshed fish (halibut, cod, etc.), cut into 1½-inch pieces

¾ pound mussels, scrubbed and debearded (ask your seafood attendant at your grocery store to handle this for you)

2 tablespoons coarsely chopped fresh parsley

In a large stockpot, heat the olive oil over medium-high heat. Add the garlic, red pepper flakes, leek, fennel, thyme, tomatoes, and bay leaves. Cook for 3 to 4 minutes, or until the vegetables are soft. Reduce the heat to medium and add the stock, clam juice, lemon juice, tomato paste, and wine. Stir to incorporate and simmer for 15 to 20 minutes.

Add the shrimp, fish, and mussels and simmer for an additional 5 minutes. Mussels should open when completely cooked. Discard any that do not open.

Right before serving, add the parsley and ladle into bowls. Enjoy!

DINNER

COMFORT MEAT LOAF

Serves: 6 to 8
Serving size: 4 ounces
Calories per serving: 234

Meat loaf is one of the best comfort foods of all time. In my version, I have swapped out ground beef for lean ground turkey. The shiitake mushrooms add a woodsy and robust flavor that marries nicely with the ground turkey. You can use portobello, cremini, or trumpet mushrooms instead of shiitakes. I turned to Swiss cheese for this recipe not only because of its mild, nutty flavor, but because it is one of the healthiest cheeses and is also available in low-fat and low-sodium versions. When you need comfort food, you can't go wrong with Comfort Meat Loaf.

1 tablespoon olive oil, plus more for greasing

1 medium red onion, finely chopped

3 garlic cloves, minced

1 cup finely chopped shiitake mushrooms

1 tablespoon Worcestershire sauce

3 tablespoons low-sodium beef stock

½ teaspoon freshly ground black pepper

1 tablespoon finely chopped fresh thyme

1 tablespoon finely chopped fresh parsley

2 large eggs, lightly beaten

¼ cup quick-cooking oats

¾ cup cubed low-fat, low-sodium Swiss cheese

1¼ pounds ground turkey breast, 99% fat-free

Preheat the oven to 400°F. Lightly oil a rimmed parchment-lined baking sheet or a 9-by-13-inch baking pan.

In a large skillet, heat the olive oil over medium heat. Add the onion and cook, stirring occasionally, until softened, about 5 minutes. Add the garlic and mushrooms and cook for about 10 minutes. Transfer the mushroom mixture to a bowl.

Add Worcestershire, beef stock, black pepper, fresh herbs, eggs, oats, and cheese to the mushroom mixture. Using your fingers, add the ground turkey and gently mix all the ingredients together to incorporate fully. The mixture will be wet, which will result in a moist meat loaf.

Form the meat loaf into a 9-by-5-inch oval, shaped like a football, and place it in the middle of the prepared pan.

Bake the meat loaf for about 45 minutes, or until it reaches an internal temperature of 170°F. Let the meat loaf stand for 5 minutes before slicing and serving.

HONEY-LEMON BAKED CHICKEN

Serves: 4
Serving size: 1 breast
Calories per serving: 201

This simple recipe bursts with tantalizing flavors, proving that healthy food can certainly please the taste buds. From the sweetness of the honey and freshness of the thyme to the acidity of the lemon, this chicken delivers on every flavor profile. Baked to perfection for a beautiful dark golden appearance and crispy texture, this is the perfect centerpiece for a weeknight meal.

2 tablespoons olive oil

1 tablespoon minced garlic

1 tablespoon lemon zest

Juice of 1 lemon

3 tablespoons honey

1 tablespoon finely chopped fresh thyme

1 teaspoon chopped fresh parsley

2 tablespoons lemon pepper seasoning with no salt

1½ teaspoons Bayou Cajun Spice Blend (page 235)

8 chicken breasts, boneless and skinless

Nonstick cooking spray

2 lemons, halved

Preheat the oven to 450°F.

In a large bowl, combine the olive oil, garlic, lemon zest, lemon juice, honey, thyme, ½ teaspoon of parsley, lemon pepper, and Bayou Cajun Spice Blend. Add the chicken to the bowl and, using your hands, coat the chicken with all the ingredients. Cover and refrigerate for 10 to 20 minutes. The longer you can let the chicken, marinate the better.

Remove the chicken from the refrigerator. Spray a baking sheet with cooking spray. Add the coated chicken to the baking sheet. Put the 4 lemon halves on each side of the baking sheet, cut-side down.

Roast the chicken for 30 to 35 minutes, or until the chicken is thoroughly cooked. Turn the pieces once during roasting. The chicken should be moist and juicy and have a crisp, dark golden color on both sides. When the chicken is done, the internal temperature of the meat will be 165°F.

Sprinkle the chicken with the remaining ½ teaspoon of parsley, and serve straight from the oven.

GRANDPA'S VEGETARIAN CHILI

Serves: 6 to 8
Serving size: 2 cups
Calories per serving: 354

Watching my grandfather make this chili inspired me to become a chef. I understood how flavors and textures worked together when I ate my favorite dish.

Don't be intimidated by the number of ingredients called for, because this one-pot wonder is super simple and cost effective and will stretch for several meals. The longer you let this chili cook, the more robust the flavor, so consider using a slow cooker.

I recommend making large batches, because this vegetarian chili freezes well. It's always great to have some delicious options in your freezer when you just don't feel like cooking.

As a time-saving tip, you can purchase prepared no-salt chili seasoning to replace the oregano, paprika, garlic powder, chili powder, and cumin.

2 tablespoons olive oil

3 garlic cloves, minced

1½ tablespoons dried oregano

1 tablespoon smoked paprika

1 tablespoon garlic powder

¼ cup chili powder

2 teaspoons ground cumin

1 small to medium Vidalia onion, chopped

1 green bell pepper, chopped

1 red bell pepper, chopped

2 (15-ounce) cans low-salt tomato sauce

1 (15-ounce) can fire-roasted tomatoes or diced tomatoes, with their liquid

2 tablespoons chopped canned chipotle chiles in adobo sauce (optional)

1 (15-ounce) can black beans, drained and rinsed

1 (15-ounce) can red kidney beans, drained and rinsed

1 cup fire-roasted corn or frozen corn

⅓ cup crushed pineapple in juice

Diced or whole jalapeño or habanero pepper to taste (optional)

2 tablespoons rice vinegar or apple cider vinegar

½ avocado, peeled and sliced

Fresh cilantro, chopped, for garnish

Scallions, thinly sliced, for garnish

In a stovetop-safe slow cooker insert or large stockpot, heat the olive oil over medium heat. Add the garlic, oregano, paprika, garlic powder, chili powder, and cumin and cook, stirring, for about 1 minute. Be careful not to burn the garlic.

Add the onion and bell peppers and cook until the peppers are soft and the onion is translucent and giving off liquid.

Add the tomato sauce, fire-roasted tomatoes, and chipotle peppers in adobo. Stir and let simmer for 2 to 3 minutes.

Add the black beans, kidney beans, corn, and pineapple. Stir over medium heat for 2 to 3 minutes.

For added heat, add jalapeño or habanero pepper.

Top it off with the vinegar. Stir and simmer over low heat for a minimum of 30 minutes. The longer you cook the chili the more intense the flavor profiles. I cook this chili for up to two hours.

Garnish with avocado slices, cilantro, and scallions.

NEW ORLEANS PECAN-CRUSTED CATFISH

Serves: 6
Serving size: 1 fillet
Calories per serving: 292

My grandfather is from New Orleans, and one of his favorite dishes is fried fish and grits. It is only fitting that I re-create the delectable taste of his favorite dish in a healthier version, because he is my inspiration for being a chef. Early on in my attempts to change my eating habits, I figured out the best way to achieve the "fried fish" effect without the deep-frying and calories. By incorporating healthy nuts with the perfect spice blend and other flavor enhancements, I cracked the code with this recipe. Get ready for some true Southern hospitality.

This recipe works with just about any type of fish. If catfish is not your cup of tea, then swap it out for halibut, cod, red snapper, swordfish, or salmon.

¾ cup finely chopped pecans

⅓ cup grated Parmigiano Reggiano cheese

4 tablespoons Bayou Cajun Spice Blend, divided (page 235; you can reduce this amount if you have sensitivity to heat)

2 tablespoons chopped fresh parsley

1 tablespoon lemon zest

1 tablespoon plus 1 teaspoon olive oil, divided

6 (5-ounce) catfish fillets, deboned

Lemon wedges, for garnish

Preheat the oven to 400°F. Line a baking sheet with parchment paper.

In a large bowl, combine the pecans, cheese, 3 tablespoons Bayou Cajun Spice Blend, parsley, lemon zest, and 1 tablespoon of the olive oil.

Place catfish fillets on the lined baking sheet. Brush the fillets with the remaining teaspoon of olive oil and rub in 1 tablespoon of the Bayou Cajun Spice Blend. Massage the oil and spice on both sides of the fish.

Spread the pecan crust liberally over the top of each piece of fish.

Bake for 15 minutes, or until the crust is dark golden and the fish is flaky and moist. Serve with lemon wedges.

STEVE HARVEY'S FAVORITE CAJUN LOBSTER MAC AND CHEESE

Serves: 6 to 8
Serving size: 1 cup
Calories per serving: 375

When I was Steve Harvey's personal chef, this was one of his favorite dishes. Now that you are in Phase 2, you get to enjoy a little pasta and cheese!

If you don't care for lobster or if you find it a bit costly, you can certainly substitute shrimp, crab meat, scallops, or, of course, chicken.

½ pound whole wheat penne

2 tablespoons olive oil

1 tablespoon minced garlic

2 tablespoons Bayou Cajun Spice Blend (page 235)

2 tablespoons flour

¼ cup finely diced red bell pepper

1 tablespoon lemon zest

2½ cups 1% milk

1 cup herbed goat cheese, at room temperature

1½ cups shredded sharp cheddar cheese

½ cup grated Parmigiano Reggiano cheese

1½ pounds lobster meat (a combination of claw, knuckle, and tail meat)

1 tablespoon chopped fresh parsley

Preheat the oven to 400°F. Put a large pot of water on to boil for the pasta.

Add the penne to the boiling water and cook according to the package directions until al dente. Drain and set aside.

In a stockpot, heat the olive oil over medium heat. Add the garlic, Bayou Cajun Spice Blend, and flour and whisk to make a roux, about 2 minutes. Adding the garlic and spice blend to the roux is my secret way to pull out the flavor.

Add the bell pepper and lemon zest and cook for 1 minute. Add the milk and whisk until the ingredients are combined. Add the goat cheese and whisk well. Allow ingredients to melt together—about 5 minutes. Add 1¼ cups of the cheddar and the Parmigiano Reggiano and whisk to combine. Simmer for 15 to 20 minutes, stirring occasionally to prevent burning. Add the lobster meat and cook for an additional 5 minutes.

Stir together the cooked pasta, cheese sauce, lobster meat, and parsley. Pour your mac and cheese into a ceramic/nonstick casserole dish or any oven-safe casserole dish and sprinkle the remaining cheddar evenly over the top. Bake for 15 to 20 minutes or until golden and bubbling.

SALADS AND SIDES

MAPLE-ROASTED SWEET POTATOES

Serves: 4
Serving size: ½ sweet potato
Calories per serving: 161

How sweet it is! You can indulge a little in Phase 2, and this dish is a perfect way to do it. The maple syrup complements the sweetness of the potatoes, the smoked paprika balances that sweetness, and the black sesame seeds are the finishing touch for texture, appearance, and flavor.

1 tablespoon olive oil

½ teaspoon smoked paprika

¼ cup pure maple syrup

⅛ teaspoon sea salt

2 sweet potatoes, peeled and cut into ½-inch wedges

2 tablespoons black sesame seeds

Preheat the oven to 400°F. Line a baking sheet with parchment paper.

In a large bowl, combine the olive oil, paprika, maple syrup, and sea salt. Add the sweet potatoes and toss until they are fully coated.

Spread the sweet potatoes in a single layer on the lined baking sheet and roast for 25 to 30 minutes, stirring gently every 5 to 10 minutes.

Sprinkle the cooked sweet potatoes with the sesame seeds. Serve hot from the oven or chilled.

ASPARAGUS MÉLANGE

Serves: 6
Serving size: At least 4 stalks
Calories per serving: 238

I love my green veggies—well, most of the time—but in my love for building ultimate flavor, I have learned how to pair my favorite green veggies with other fruits and vegetables to deliver harmonious taste profiles. One thing you will experience from this recipe and the others in this book is how every dish or meal will satisfy most, if not all, of the senses on your palate—sweet, salty, spicy, savory, bitter, and sour.

I pound asparagus, ends removed about I inch from the bottom

2 tablespoons chopped fresh basil

¼ cup extra-virgin olive oil

Juice of I lime

I teaspoon Dijon mustard

I teaspoon freshly ground black pepper

¼ cup thinly sliced shallots

I pound cherry tomatoes

½ cup I-inch cubes fresh pineapple

2 large ripe avocados, pitted, peeled, and cut into large cubes

Bring a pot of water to boil. Fill a large bowl with ice and water and have it nearby. Add the asparagus and boil for 1 to 2 minutes. Quickly remove the asparagus from the boiling water and transfer them to the ice water to stop the cooking, a technique called shocking. Let the asparagus sit in the ice water for 5 to 10 minutes or until completely cooled and bright green in color. Cut the asparagus into 2-inch pieces.

In a large bowl, combine the basil, olive oil, lime juice, mustard, pepper, and shallots. Whisk until well mixed. Add the asparagus, cherry tomatoes, pineapple, and avocado. Gently toss to combine fully.

SPICED KALE AND COCONUT QUINOA STIR-FRY

Serves: 4
Serving size: 1 cup
Calories per serving: 317

The combination of kale and quinoa makes this a very nutritious vegetarian main course. As a side, it certainly flavors up a dinner plate.

Stir-fries are excellent weekday dinners, because you can whip them up in no time at all. You can add strips of chicken, pork, or beef, or shrimp or scallops to up the protein. Building a stir-fry is a great opportunity to combine flavors. Have fun creating your own flavor combinations.

2 tablespoons olive oil, divided

2 large eggs, beaten

3 garlic cloves, minced

¾ cup chopped scallions

½ cup bean sprouts

¾ cup unsweetened coconut flakes

1 bunch lacinato kale or curly kale, stemmed, leaves shredded

2 cups cooked quinoa

1 tablespoon low-sodium soy sauce

2 teaspoons chile-garlic sauce

1 teaspoon Sriracha

Juice of 1 lime

2 tablespoons fresh whole Thai basil leaves (optional)

Heat a large skillet or wok over medium-high heat. Add 1 teaspoon of the olive oil and the beaten eggs to the wok. Stir continuously to scramble the eggs until cooked, about 2 minutes. Transfer the eggs to a bowl.

Add the remaining oil to the pan along with the garlic, scallions, bean sprouts, coconut, kale, and quinoa. Cook for 3 minutes. Return the egg to the skillet. Add the soy sauce, chile-garlic sauce, Sriracha, and lime. Gently fold all the ingredients together. Garnish with the Thai basil and serve.

SWEET POTATO CRUMBLE

Serves: 4 to 6
Serving size: 1 cup
Calories per serving: 358

Sweet Potato Crumble is the perfect holiday "mash-up," where candied yams meet Grandma's sweet potato pie. This ideal holiday side dish gets healthy while still delivering nostalgic flavors. I use avocado, almond milk, and roasted sweet potatoes for a decadent base and infuse sweetness with dates and pineapple.

Instead of a traditional piecrust, the recipe creates a textural element with an oatmeal, raisin, and caramelized pecan crumble on top to take this dish to the next level.

FOR THE SWEET POTATO BASE:

7 medium sweet potatoes

¼ cup fresh ripe pineapple, finely chopped

2 tablespoons honey

3 tablespoons pure maple syrup

1½ tablespoons pure vanilla extract

1 teaspoon ground cinnamon

½ teaspoon ground nutmeg

1 avocado, pitted and peeled

½ cup unsweetened vanilla almond milk

FOR THE CRUMBLE TOPPING:

½ cup old-fashioned rolled oats

1 tablespoon honey

1½ teaspoons flour

½ teaspoon ground cinnamon

¼ cup finely chopped pecans

2 tablespoons dried unsweetened cranberries

2 tablespoons raisins

1½ teaspoons olive oil

Make the sweet potato base: Preheat the oven to 400°F.

Wrap each potato in aluminum foil and place them on a baking sheet. Roast for about 60 minutes, or until soft. Let cool for 10 to 15 minutes. Separate the sweet potato flesh from the skin, and place the flesh in a bowl. Using a potato masher, coarsely mash the potatoes. Stir in the pineapple, honey, maple syrup, vanilla, cinnamon, and nutmeg.

In a blender, combine the avocado and almond milk and blend until thick, smooth, and creamy. Transfer the avocado mixture to the bowl with the potatoes and fold together. Pour the sweet potato mixture into a ceramic or nonstick baking dish.

Make the crumble topping: In a separate bowl, combine the oats, honey, flour, cinnamon, pecans, cranberries, raisins, and olive oil and stir. Sprinkle the crumble on top of the sweet potato mixture.

Bake for 25 to 30 minutes, or until golden brown and bubbling.

DESSERTS

EARL GREY–INFUSED LEMON GRANITA

Serves: 4 to 6
Serving size: 1 cup
Calories per serving: 90

Imagine tea with lemon turned into a coarse sorbet. That's what granita is, and it is a breeze to make. It takes high tea to a new level!

I tablespoon loose Earl Grey tea, in an infuser, or I Earl Grey tea bag

I teaspoon lemon zest, plus more for garnish

½ cup fresh lemon juice (from about 3 lemons)

½ cup raw honey

In a small pot, bring 4 cups of water to a boil. Remove from the heat and add the tea. Steep for 4 minutes. Remove the tea from the liquid and let it cool for up to 10 minutes. Add the lemon zest, lemon juice, and honey and stir until all the ingredients have dissolved. Refrigerate for 45 minutes.

Transfer to a freezer-friendly container with a lid and freeze for 1 hour. Remove from the freezer and break up the ice that has formed at the top with a fork. Return to the freezer and repeat the breaking of the ice every hour for 2 to 3 hours, until the granita is flaky and uniformly frozen.

Serve by scraping out the granita with a spoon and garnishing with lemon zest.

CHOCOLATE BANANA BITES

Yields 8 bites
Serving size: 3 pieces
Calories per serving: 100

This recipe is super simple and healthy, and will satisfy anyone's discerning sweet tooth. Keep in mind that bananas are a real power food—a type of healthy carbohydrate that helps you burn calories and eat less. These bites are so good, you have to be mindful of your portion size!

2 tablespoons dark chocolate chips	I teaspoon honey
½ teaspoon ground espresso beans(optional)	I large banana, cut into I-inch pieces

Place the chocolate chips, espresso, and honey in a microwave-safe bowl. Microwave for 1 to 1½ minutes, or until chocolate has melted.

Stir to combine fully.

Dip half of each 1-inch banana piece in the chocolate, set on a plate lined with parchment paper, and refrigerate to set the chocolate. This dessert is also amazing frozen.

GUILTLESS LEMON-BLUEBERRY CAKE MILK SHAKE

Serves: 2
Serving Size: 1 cup
Calories per serving: 142

This milk shake does not disappoint, offering all the flavor and decadence of a traditional shake without all the fat, sugar, and calories. Infusing two summer favorites—lemon and blueberries—makes for a perfect marriage. Substituting frozen bananas and avocado for heavy cream is a smart diet strategy. This recipe uses a banana to achieve a creamy texture.

This milk shake is wonderful as a morning beverage as well as a dessert. You can drink this guiltless milk shake with a straw or eat it with a spoon.

⅔ cup unsweetened almond milk

¼ cup light coconut milk

½ cup frozen blueberries

1 cup cubed frozen banana

½ teaspoon lemon zest

1 tablespoon fresh lemon juice

½ teaspoon pure vanilla extract

1 teaspoon honey

2 tablespoons crushed reduced-fat
    vanilla wafer cookies (optional)

In a high-powered blender, combine all the ingredients except the vanilla wafer cookies and lemon zest. Hold back a few blueberries for garnish. Blend until thick, rich, and creamy.

Top with fresh lemon zest, blueberries, and the crushed vanilla wafer cookies if you'd like.

GRANDMA'S CARROT CAKE OATMEAL COOKIES

Yield: 12 to 14 cookies
Serving Size: 1 cookie
Calories per serving: 122

My grandmother was the queen of baking, and carrot cake was one of her favorites to make. Needless to say, it quickly became one of my favorites to eat! Although Grandma had no shame using lots of butter and sugar, I decided to pay homage to her with a healthier, bite-size version of her classic cake.

This recipe makes a bunch of cookies, but don't feel tempted to double dip into the cookie jar! These cookies freeze wonderfully. Wrap each cookie in a small baggie, place them in a large sealable plastic bag, and freeze. When you desire something sweet, you'll be able to enjoy one of these low-calorie cookies to satisfy your craving.

If you have a nut allergy, omit the walnuts and substitute sunflower or chia seeds.

Nonstick cooking spray

¾ cup whole wheat flour

1 cup instant oats

1½ teaspoons baking powder

2 teaspoons ground cinnamon

¼ teaspoon ground nutmeg

⅛ teaspoon kosher salt

2 tablespoons coconut oil, melted

1 large egg, at room temperature

1 tablespoon pure vanilla extract

½ cup pure maple syrup

¾ cup grated carrots

2 tablespoons finely chopped walnuts

¼ cup golden raisins

Preheat the oven to 325°F. Line a baking sheet with parchment paper and spray with cooking spray.

In a large bowl, combine the flour, oats, baking powder, cinnamon, nutmeg, and salt. In a separate bowl, combine the coconut oil, egg, and vanilla and whisk to incorporate. Add the maple syrup and stir to mix fully. Add the dry ingredients and stir to combine. Gently fold in the carrots, walnuts, and raisins. Cover the bowl with plastic wrap and refrigerate for 25 to 30 minutes.

Scoop the dough into 1½-inch balls and line them up on the prepared baking sheet, leaving enough room for the cookies to spread. Bake for 12 to 15 minutes. Transfer the cookies to a plate. Let them cool for up to 10 minutes before eating.

DECADENT CHOCOLATE PEANUT BUTTER CUP "ICE CREAM"

Serves: 2 to 4
Serving size: ½ cup
Calories per serving: 175

I call this "ice cream" decadent for a reason—it's that creamy and delicious! It's hard to believe what a caloric bargain it is. Sometimes even a couple of teaspoons of this dessert is enough to satisfy my sweet cravings.

2 or 3 overripe bananas, peeled and frozen

1 tablespoon no-sugar-added natural peanut butter (creamy or chunky)

1 teaspoon pure vanilla extract

⅛ teaspoon ground cardamom

2 tablespoons raw honey

2 tablespoons dark chocolate chips

Put the frozen bananas in a food processor and puree, scraping down the sides periodically, until the bananas are rich and smooth in consistency. Add the peanut butter, vanilla, cardamom, and honey and puree.

Transfer the "ice cream" from the food processor to a freezer-friendly dish or container. Fold in the chocolate chips and freeze for up to 3 hours. Enjoy one scoop of this deliciousness!!

I hope my recipes inspire you to play with flavor in your own kitchen. I want you to feel empowered to put together your own combinations of flavors and ingredients, and to get comfortable whipping up your own delicious meals and snacks based on what you're most excited to eat. With that in mind, I have created twenty-five spice blends that will add instant flavor to your food and give you a shortcut for preparing delicious meals. The spice blends re-create flavor profiles from around the world. I want to make turning out delicious meals quick and easy. No bland food should come from your kitchen again!

11

SPICE BLENDS FOR INSTANT FLAVOR

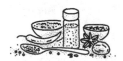

Let's face it—there are some evenings you have absolutely no interest in coming home, opening a cookbook, and figuring out what to make. Even as a chef, I get it, but don't let an off night derail your new healthy lifestyle. I have created twenty-five of my favorite spice blends for you to use whenever your meal has to be fast and easy and, of course, taste insanely delicious. You can sprinkle these on some plain, basic ingredients to instantly transform them into something special. Even when you're short on time and can't cook a full recipe, these blends are the foundation for making any meal scrumptious in as much time as you have. The rest is simple.

You have been using spices in the recipes for Phases 1 and 2, but this chapter will take your spice knowledge up a notch and show you how to customize any recipe. In this chapter you will find recipes for well-balanced flavor profiles of blended spices that will make healthy food mouth-watering and fun. Once you are comfortable using these blends, cooking will become an adventure of your choosing that can take you anywhere in the world.

You can make batches of the blends to store in airtight jars away from direct light, heat, and humidity to preserve the freshness of the spices and herbs. Kept this way, your spice blends should last about a year. If you store your blends in the refrigerator or freezer, make sure they are in an airtight container or plastic bag, because condensation can form when you take them out. The condensation can cause oxidation, which results in quick flavor loss, as I explained on page 123. You can store the blends in good-looking mason jars with airtight lids. Some other storage solutions that might work for you include keeping your spices in a kitchen drawer or using a decorative box that complements your kitchen. Have fun using creative and interesting labels on the storage jars. With these prepared spice blends waiting for you, you will be able to make palate-pleasing meals in a snap. As you get familiar with how spices work together, you can move on to creating original blends for your own kitchen or to share with friends. When you make your own blends, you can have fun getting innovative in naming the flavor profile.

Like a Kid in a Candy Store

The spice blends we were able to design during the Blue Cross Blue Shield of Illinois program was like me being a kid in a candy store. My favorite was the Dill Pickle Spice Blend. I worked with spices and ingredients I had never used before. When I got home, I paired them with Chef Judson's recommendations. They were fabulous. I can't wait for *The Spice Diet* book to hit the shelves, because I now consider myself a healthier foodie! I am so ready to lose weight and keep it off forever!

—*Anne M.*

HOW MY SPICE BLENDS CAN MAKE YOU A SUPERSTAR IN THE KITCHEN

I started creating the spice blends for myself. After crazy days cooking for others, I often want to throw something simple together to eat. I play no games when it comes to my food and serious flavor, and these spice blends give me everything I need. As you become familiar with the spices and blends, be conservative with the amount you use until you know the impact of the flavor on your food and your palate. I use the blends for spiced-up snacks, dressings, dips, main dishes, and much more. The following suggestions will show you how to put the spice blends to good use:

- Sprinkled on raw "healthier" nuts, such as almonds, pecans, pistachios, and cashews, which I roast on a baking sheet in a 350°F oven for snacks. It takes no more than 5 minutes. I add some dried cherries and golden raisins, and I am in a crunchy, sweet, and savory euphoria—with no interest in being brought back to reality. I make a lot at a time and store my spiced nuts in a tightly covered jar or plastic container. I must admit that I have to portion these jewels in small plastic bags, so I don't overindulge. Here's a little secret: You can take them with you to work or carry a bag with you when you are out and about. You can keep a bag in your glove compartment for an emergency snack to hold you over until you get home to your choice of healthy foods.

- Sprinkle a blend you like on freshly popped popcorn for an added flavor kick.

- The spice blends enliven salad dressings. Just mix one part vinegar or fresh lemon juice with four parts of extra-virgin olive oil in a jar, add about 1 teaspoon of spice blend, then seal the jar and shake it up. The oil in the dressing releases the flavors of the spices. Be sure to taste test the dressing. It's better to start using the blends conservatively and adding more to reach the flavor blast you want. This salad dressing will keep in your refrigerator for up to 2 weeks. If you use dairy, preferably nonfat Greek yogurt, or fresh vegetable purees like cauliflower or avocado in the dressing, the dressing should keep for up to a week. Don't forget to also work in a "foodie's" best friend—garlic—as well as fresh herbs like thyme, dill, parsley, mint, and chives in any combination.

- You can make tasty dips with the spice blends. Mix some into nonfat yogurt or plain hummus, and you have a tasty dip for raw vegetables or kale chips.

ONE OF MY FAVORITE DIPS

½ cup low-fat Greek yogurt

1 tablespoon Jamaican Me Crazy Jerk Seasoning (recipe follows)

1 tablespoon chopped scallion

1 teaspoon fresh lime juice

Combine all the ingredients in a bowl and stir well to incorporate. I enjoy this spicy, savory, rich and creamy dip with baked plantain chips or other roast veggies.

- You can mix a blend with low-sodium chicken, beef, or vegetable stock to use as a base for soup.

- I sprinkle spice blends on steamed vegetables that have been tossed with a touch of olive oil or grapeseed oil. Using a spice blend on roasted vegetables also adds a flavor kick. Put pieces of broccoli or cauliflower, halved Brussels sprouts, carrot chips, or whatever vegetable you are using in a plastic bag and shake the veggies up with a bit of olive oil until they are coated. Remember that a little oil acts as a flavor releaser. Put the vegetables on a parchment-lined baking sheet, which will save you cleanup time, and sprinkle your spice blend of choice on the veggies. You can sprinkle the vegetables with a spice blend before or after you roast them. When you roast the vegetables with the spice blend and oil, the spices cook with the veggies and produce a more pronounced, deeper flavor. Roast in a 375°F oven for 30 to 45 minutes, depending on how crispy you like your vegetables. When you take the pan out of the oven, taste a piece of veggie and sprinkle it with a bit more spice blend if needed. I roast vegetables in large quantities, because they make great snacks. I store them in a covered container on the counter or in the refrigerator, depending on how quickly I eat them. They are my replacement for greasy, salty chips.

- Spice blends make delicious dry rubs. Pat a blend liberally on meat, poultry, or fish before cooking. Score the meat lightly, which means to cut small gashes in the surface of the meat, so that the flavors penetrate more deeply. The amount of time you should refrigerate the rubbed meat before cooking depends on how strong the flavor of the spice blend is. More powerful blends require less time. Marinating time varies from 15 minutes to several hours. For heightened flavor, let your meat marinate overnight. It's up to you and the amount of time you have.

- You can make a wet rub, or paste, by adding the spice blend to a moist ingredient. You might try yogurt, mustard, finely chopped garlic, horseradish, or olive oil. A wet rub will stick to the food more easily. Sometimes I brush a small amount of oil on a piece of fish, sprinkle on some spice blend, and bake, broil, or grill the fish.

- To make a traditional marinade, mix ¼ cup water, ¼ cup vinegar or lemon juice, ¼ cup olive oil, and a little more than 1 tablespoon spice blend. You might want to add 1 teaspoon chopped garlic. Coat the meat you are cooking with the mixture and let it marinate, covered, in the refrigerator. Poultry and fish need less time marinating than meat. Meat needs at least 1 hour to overnight to marinate for the best flavor. Poultry and fish require only about 15 minutes.

- The spice blends add flavor to simple, healthy sauces.

AN "ALL-PURPOSE" HEALTHY CREAM SAUCE

Yield: 2 cups

This recipe for a simple sauce, which doesn't use cream or butter, will become one of your go-to recipes. This basic recipe transfers to many sauces, because you can use the spice blend of your choice for flavor.

1½ tablespoons olive oil

1 tablespoon Bayou Cajun Spice Blend (page 235) or your favorite spice blend

1 tablespoon minced garlic

⅓ cup unsweetened coconut milk or skim milk

2 cups white wine

1 tablespoon water

½ teaspoon lemon zest

1 tablespoon cornstarch

In a small saucepot, heat the oil over medium-low heat. Add the spice blend and garlic and cook for 2 minutes.

Whisk in the milk, wine, and lemon zest.

In a separate bowl, whisk together 1 tablespoon water and the cornstarch, making sure there are no lumps, to make a slurry. Whisk the cornstarch slurry into the sauce to thicken it. Your end result should be a beautiful, slightly thick sauce.

SPICE BLEND RECIPES

I have created twenty-five of my signature spice blends that are simple to make and will add bold flavor dimension to everything you cook. No more bland and tired food!

The spice blends are divided into three groups. The first are foundational recipes, which are basic and can be used to replace salt and to flavor soups, meat, poultry, seafood, and vegetables. The next category, The United States of Flavor, covers our rich variety of regional foods—from N'awlins Spiced Pecan Crust Blend to Little Italy Blend to Sour Dill Pickle Blend. Finally, the Global blends are your passport to a flavor excursion around the world—from Japan to Mexico to Greece. Add these exotic flavor profiles to your cooking and you will never be bored with healthy food again.

You will be using dried spices and herbs in all the spice blend recipes, unless otherwise indicated. I have deliberately avoided using seeds that you would have to crush in a mortar and pestle or spice grinder to prepare. At this point, I want to streamline the process for you. Sticking to the pre-ground versions of some seeds will save you time. As you get more sophisticated, you might want to experiment with grinding your own spices and herbs.

FOUNDATIONAL

These are basic blends for specific purposes, with the exception of the seasoned salt substitute, which you will find yourself using on everything. From soup to chicken to veggies, these blends will win a permanent place in your repertoire for adding flavor to everyday meals.

SALT-FREE BETTER-THAN-SALT BLEND

Yield: about ⅔ cup

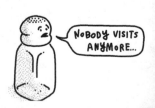

If your diet has consisted of processed and fast food, you should consider seriously limiting your salt intake. If you have hypertension, you have to cut back significantly on the amount of salt you eat for your health. So many people salt their food before they have even tasted it, which can mask the natural flavor of the food. This blend will enhance the flavor of everything you use it on.

2 tablespoons dried basil

2 tablespoons dried parsley

2 tablespoons dried chives

2 tablespoons dried savory

2 teaspoons ground rosemary

2 teaspoons sweet paprika

2 teaspoons granulated onion

1½ tablespoons powdered milk

Mix all the ingredients together thoroughly in an airtight container and store away from heat and light.

SAVORY SOUP SPICE BLEND

Yield: ½ cup

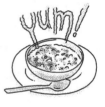

Simply add this soup blend to chicken, beef, or veggie stock to create a base for a tasty soup. Toss in any veggies, chicken, or seafood you like.

2 tablespoons dried parsley

1 tablespoon dried thyme

1 tablespoon granulated garlic

1½ teaspoons dried chervil

1½ teaspoons dried basil

1½ teaspoons dried marjoram

1½ teaspoons dried celery seed

1 teaspoon dried savory

1 teaspoon dried rosemary

1 teaspoon fresh or dried lemon zest*

Mix all the ingredients together thoroughly in an airtight container. Store away from heat and light at room temperature if you use dried lemon zest, and in the freezer in a tightly sealed plastic bag if you use fresh zest.

*Use a Microplane grater or zester if you are using fresh lemon zest. All the natural flavor and oils exist in the skin of citrus.

POULTRY SPICE BLEND

Yield: a little more than 2 tablespoons

You will be eating a lot of chicken as a source of lean protein on the Spice Diet. This blend will make your poultry anything but bland. Get ready for a feast for your taste buds. Make sure you have leftovers, because the chicken will be incredible, seared or grilled and added to a veggie bowl or mixed with lime-infused avocado, roasted corn, and fresh cherry tomatoes. Cold leftover chicken is delicious in a salad or a wrap.

2 teaspoons ground mace

½ teaspoon dried sage

1½ teaspoons dried thyme

1 teaspoon dried marjoram

¾ teaspoon dried rosemary

½ teaspoon ground nutmeg

½ teaspoon ground black pepper

Mix together all the ingredients in an airtight container and store in a cool, dry place.

VEGGIES NEVER TASTED LIKE THIS BLEND

Yield: 1 cup

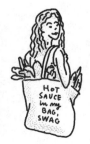

If you are like most Americans, you do not eat enough vegetables. They are the source of so many vital vitamins and minerals, and the value of the fiber they contain should not be underestimated when it comes to weight loss and overall health. When you sprinkle this blend over your vegetables, you will eat all your veggies first. I know I do.

5 tablespoons dried parsley	I tablespoon dried marjoram
I tablespoon dried oregano	I tablespoon granulated garlic
2½ tablespoons paprika	I½ teaspoons dried savory
2 tablespoons celery seed	I teaspoon dried thyme
2 teaspoons cayenne pepper	I teaspoon chili powder
I tablespoon ground mustard	

Mix together all the ingredients in an airtight container and store in a cool, dry place away from heat and light.

UNITED STATES OF FLAVOR

American regional food is exceptionally varied. I have captured some of my favorite regional and ethnic flavors in these spice blends.

N'AWLINS SPICED PECAN CRUST BLEND

Yield: 1½ cups

If you didn't already know, I love a good piece of fried fish, but I know it's not something I can add to my daily food intake. This spice blend was created to take my insatiable love for fried fish to a much healthier and tastier level.

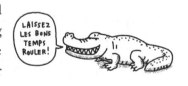

If crunch is your thing, this Cajun crust has rich flavor and great texture. It's a wonderful substitute for the batter or bread crumbs usually used to coat chicken or fish for deep-frying.

All you have to do is brush the protein with a little olive oil and sprinkle the N'awlins Spiced Pecan Crust Blend liberally to coat the top for fish or chicken. The oil helps the crust stick to your protein. You can bake the chicken or fish in a 400°F oven. The fish should take about 10 minutes, depending on how thick the piece is. Test it with a fork to see if it is flaky and moist. Chicken with the bone in will take longer than boneless chicken breasts or thighs. At 375°F, the chicken should cook for about 30 minutes or until it reaches an internal temperature of 165°F.

I cup pecans, finely chopped (crushed or pulsed in a blender or food processor to desired texture)

2 tablespoons finely chopped fresh parsley

½ teaspoon fresh lemon zest

I tablespoon Bayou Cajun Spice Blend (page 235)

Mix all the ingredients together in a resealable plastic bag or airtight container. Store in the freezer.

SPECIAL "FRIED" CHICKEN

olive oil

chicken

Bayou Cajun Spice Blend (page 235)

egg, beaten

N'awlins Spiced Pecan Crust Blend (page 229)

Preheat the oven to 350°F.

Brush olive oil on both sides of a piece of chicken. Sprinkle Bayou Cajun Spice Blend on both sides.

Dip the chicken in the egg wash.

Coat the chicken with the N'awlins Spiced Pecan Crust Blend.

Bake for 30 to 40 minutes for boneless chicken breasts and thighs and 45 to 60 minutes for bone-in chicken. The internal temperature of the chicken should be 165°F. For bone-in chicken, the chicken should no longer be pink at the bone and the juices should run clear. Turn once during baking so that the chicken pieces have uniform color and crunch.

NUTS 4 ALMOND COCONUT CRUST BLEND

Yield: about 1⅓ cups

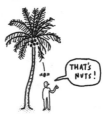

This is a versatile crust blend that will add exotic flavor and crunchy, moist texture to any meat. To use, brush your protein—lean pork tenderloin or a piece of fish like cod or halibut are great—with olive oil, then pat the crust on and put the pan in the oven. It's like eating a candy bar without the chocolate. It also pairs nicely with chicken and lamb.

¾ cup almonds, finely chopped in a blender or food processor

½ cup unsweetened shredded coconut, toasted

Honey

Brush the protein you are cooking with olive oil, then liberally sprinkle the crust on top. Drizzle the top of each piece of protein with a very small amount of honey. The honey is not part of the crust, but it pairs with the crust for a sweet flavor profile.

LITTLE ITALY SPICE BLEND

Yield: about ½ cup

If you mix this blend into lean ground beef or turkey, you can make perfect meatballs or meat loaf and your own Italian dressing with much more depth than one that comes in a bottle. When you are in Phase 2 and can eat whole wheat pasta, all you have to do is toss a teaspoon of this blend with a little olive oil and a cup of cooked whole wheat pasta for a side dish for two. It also pairs nicely with pasta, red sauce, chicken, veal, and fish.

3 tablespoons dried oregano

3 tablespoons dried basil

1½ teaspoons dried minced garlic

¼ teaspoon red pepper flakes

Mix together all the ingredients in an airtight container and store in a cool, dry place away from heat and light.

SOUR DILL PICKLE SPICE BLEND

Yield: about ⅓ cup

Dill and lemon is a familiar combination, and the garlic in this blend adds another layer of flavor. I use it on salmon and delicate fish like sole or flounder. This blend is not overpowering. It's great in a broth-based soup. It also pairs well with shellfish.

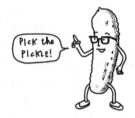

2 tablespoons dried dill

3 tablespoons lemon pepper

1 teaspoon granulated garlic

Mix all the ingredients in an airtight container and store in a cool, dry place away from heat and light.

GRANDDAD'S BBQ SPICE BLEND

Yield: about 1⅓ cups

Watching my grandfather cook taught me about layering flavor. You will never want to pour barbecue sauce from a bottle again after you season your food with this blend. Rub it on chicken, pork, steak, a hamburger, skewered shrimp, a veggie burger, or a roast and you will taste barbecue as you have never had it before. It's also great on vegetables.

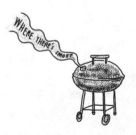

½ cup packed brown sugar

½ cup paprika

1 tablespoon ground black pepper

1 tablespoon chili powder

1 tablespoon garlic powder

1 tablespoon onion powder

2 teaspoons mustard powder

1 teaspoon cayenne pepper

Mix together all the ingredients in an airtight container and store in a cool, dry place away from heat and light.

CHESAPEAKE BAY CRAB AND SEAFOOD SPICE BLEND

Yield: ½ cup

Although this type of spice blend originated in Maryland by the Chesapeake Bay, it has become popular in all the Middle Atlantic States, New England, the Gulf Coast, and the South. I do a quick shrimp boil using this blend. There's nothing like a pile of peel-and-eat shrimp for a feast!

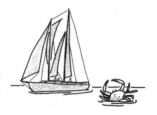

You don't have to stick to seafood. There are a million ways to use this blend—sprinkled on eggs, salads, popcorn, dips, rubbed on a chicken for roasting or grilling.

2 tablespoons ground bay leaves	I teaspoon ground nutmeg
2 tablespoons celery salt	I teaspoon ground cloves
I tablespoon dry mustard	I teaspoon ground allspice
2 teaspoons ground black pepper	½ teaspoon red pepper flakes
2 teaspoons ground ginger	½ teaspoon ground mace
2 teaspoons sweet paprika	½ teaspoon ground cardamom
I teaspoon ground white pepper	¼ teaspoon ground cinnamon

Mix together all the ingredients in an airtight container and store in a cool, dry place away from heat and light.

TEX-MEX CHILI SPICE BLEND

Yield: ¼ cup

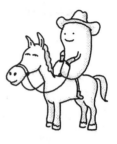

A perennial favorite, chili is versatile because you can serve it with so many toppings: chopped tomatoes, onion, avocados, jalapeños, bell peppers, and grated cheese like cheddar, Monterey Jack, or a four-cheese Mexican blend. Talk about flavor and texture! You can use chopped chicken, beef, turkey, or vegetables as a base. See page 208 for a terrific chili recipe.

1 tablespoon yellow cornmeal	½ teaspoon granulated garlic
1½ teaspoons chili powder	½ teaspoon ground cumin
½ teaspoon red pepper flakes, crushed	1 teaspoon dried oregano
2 tablespoons dried onion powder	½ teaspoon ground ancho chile

Mix together all the ingredients in an airtight container and store in a cool, dry place away from heat and light.

BLACKENED SPICE BLEND

Yield: ¼ cup

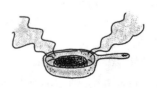

"Blackened" is a Cajun method of cooking fish, meat, or poultry by searing it over very high heat in a cast-iron skillet. The protein ends up charred and the spice blend adds an extra punch. I am supplying you with a basic recipe for a blackening spice blend. You can experiment and add other spices to this mixture. It pairs well with fish, chicken, and beef.

1 tablespoon kosher salt	1 tablespoon paprika
2 teaspoons freshly ground black pepper	1 teaspoon dried thyme
1 tablespoon cayenne pepper	1 teaspoon dried oregano

Mix together all the ingredients in an airtight container and store in a cool, dry place away from heat and light.

SUNSHINE CITRUS SPICE BLEND

Yield: ⅓ cup

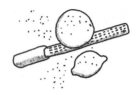

This blend puts a smile on my face just thinking about it. The light citrus makes the flavor of this blend sparkle, the nutmeg grounds the flavor, the ginger and garlic add pungency, the red pepper heats it up, and the parsley amalgamates the flavors. This blend can be used on just about anything: fish, shellfish, chicken, vegetables, pasta, soups, sauces, and marinades.

- 1 tablespoon ground nutmeg
- 1 tablespoon ground ginger
- 1 tablespoon orange zest, dried or fresh
- 1 teaspoon lemon zest, dried or fresh
- 1 teaspoon granulated garlic
- 1 teaspoon red pepper flakes
- 1 teaspoon dried parsley

Mix together all the ingredients. Store in an airtight container in the freezer if you use fresh zest or in a cool, dry place away from heat and light if you use dried zest.

BAYOU CAJUN SPICE BLEND

Yield: ¼ cup

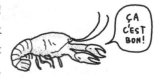

Cajun cuisine is the food of my ancestors! I love it. Let the good times roll! When I think about catfish now, I think about this blend. It works well with any white-fleshed fish, shrimp, or poultry, and brings vegetables to life.

2 teaspoons freshly ground white pepper

2 teaspoons garlic powder

2 teaspoons onion powder

2 teaspoons cayenne pepper

2 teaspoons paprika

1 tablespoon dried thyme

2 teaspoons ground black pepper

½ teaspoon mustard powder

Mix together all the ingredients in an airtight container and store in a cool, dry place away from heat and light.

GLOBAL

I have traveled widely and studied exotic flavor profiles from all over the globe. I am fascinated to learn the spice combinations that capture the tastes and aromas of countries around the world. Because we are a melting pot in the United States, a multitude of cultures are represented in the food and ingredients available to us, and not just in big cities. You will enjoy these flavor profiles from Mexico, Japan, Thailand, and Morocco, to name just a few. To get super creative and trendy, try making up your own global fusion cuisine using the various blends. My favorite global flavor "mash-ups" are Thai and Creole blends.

FIESTA SPICE BLEND

Yield: a little more than ½ cup

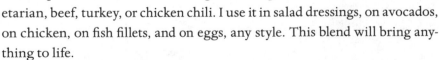

LET'S SPICE THINGS UP!

Mexican food is my favorite, so I use the Fiesta Spice Blend all the time. It's great in vegetarian, beef, turkey, or chicken chili. I use it in salad dressings, on avocados, on chicken, on fish fillets, and on eggs, any style. This blend will bring anything to life.

¼ cup chili powder

2 tablespoons paprika

1 tablespoon onion powder

1 tablespoon garlic powder

1 teaspoon red pepper flakes

1 tablespoon ground cumin

1 teaspoon fresh lime zest

Mix together all the ingredients in an airtight container and store in the freezer.

ZESTY PARMESAN SPICE BLEND

Yield: 2 cups

No longer considered exotic, Italian cuisine is the most popular in this country. If you want to visit sunny Italy—at least with your taste buds—just sprinkle this blend on vegetables or use it as a coating for chicken or the flavor base for salad dressing.

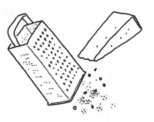

¾ cup grated Parmigiano Reggiano cheese (6 ounces)

3 tablespoons dried Italian seasoning (such as the Little Italy Spice Blend, page 231)

3 tablespoons dried parsley

1 tablespoon garlic powder

½ teaspoon red pepper flakes

1 tablespoon lemon pepper seasoning (no salt added)

Mix together all the ingredients in an airtight container and store in the freezer.

JAMAICAN ME CRAZY JERK SPICE BLEND

Yield: about ⅓ cup

When you want to escape to a Caribbean Island, just put on some reggae and use this jerk spice blend. Its pungent flavor will remind you of white sand and turquoise water even in the dead of winter. While the flavors will transport you to the islands, we all know, for the full experience, you are going to have to book that much-needed vacation. This blend pairs nicely with chicken, pork, and seafood.

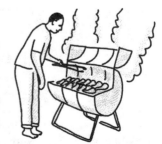

2 teaspoons ground allspice	2 tablespoons granulated garlic
1 tablespoon dried thyme	2 teaspoons cracked black pepper
1 teaspoon red pepper flakes	1½ teaspoons onion powder

Mix together all the ingredients in an airtight container and store in a cool, dry place away from heat and light.

JAPANESE-INSPIRED SPICE BLEND

Yield: about 3 tablespoons

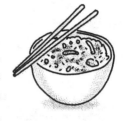

If the salt in Japanese foods and sauces gets to you, this blend is a healthy way to reproduce the flavor you love. I make a marinade with this blend and marinate shrimp in it for about 10 minutes in the refrigerator, then grill the shrimp on skewers. This blend works well sprinkled over steamed vegetables that have been lightly tossed with olive oil. You won't have trouble eating more vegetables when they taste like this. It pairs nicely with fish, shellfish, and vegetarian dishes.

½ sheet nori (dried seaweed), chopped in a blender or food processor	2 teaspoons sesame seeds
	½ teaspoon ground ginger
1 teaspoon red pepper flakes	1 teaspoon granulated garlic

Mix together all the ingredients in an airtight container and store in a cool, dry place away from heat and light.

INDIAN MASALA SPICE BLEND

Yield: ⅓ cup

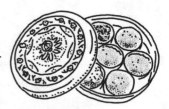

When you make your own tandoori masala spice blend, you will probably find that layers of flavor exist that you never have tasted before. Giving a nod to the flavors of India, this blend works well mixed in yogurt as a dip, in quinoa with vegetables, and in a sauce with light coconut milk or yogurt. This blend also pairs well with chicken, beef, pork, lamb, shellfish, and vegetables.

⅓ teaspoon ground fenugreek seeds

1 teaspoon ground coriander

3 to 7 teaspoons smoked paprika

1 teaspoon ground cumin

½ teaspoon ground cloves

½ teaspoon ground cardamom

½ teaspoon ground cinnamon

1 teaspoon ground turmeric

1½ teaspoons ground ginger

¾ teaspoon cayenne pepper

1 teaspoon garam masala

Mix together all the ingredients in an airtight container and store in a cool, dry place away from heat and light.

YEAR OF THE DRAGON SPICE MARINADE

Yield: about 1 cup

You can whip up a meal in no time at all if you use a wok and stir-fry strips of meat with vegetables. You do not need to use a lot of oil. Once the food is prepped, the cooking time is speedy. Just begin your stir-fry with this marinade and you will have a delicious meal.

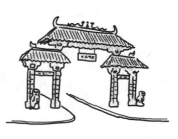

By adding coconut oil, fresh garlic and ginger, lime juice, and seafood stock, this spice blend can be used as a sauce for a stir-fry or as a marinade for veggies, fish, pork, chicken, or even tofu. If you have more time, you can marinate any sort of protein to get that unmistakable Chinese flavor without the MSG. It pairs well with chicken, beef, pork, fish, shellfish, and vegetarian dishes.

½ cup low-sodium soy sauce

2 tablespoons sesame oil

3 tablespoons honey

½ teaspoon red pepper flakes

½ teaspoon ground ginger

1 tablespoon garlic powder

1 tablespoon Chinese five-spice powder

Mix together all the ingredients in an airtight container and store in the refrigerator for up to 1 week.

THAI SPICE BLEND

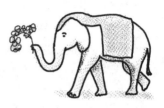

Yield: about ½ cup

I'm wild about Thai food, because the flavors are very bold. Thai food melds opposites very successfully. Fiery curry paste is paired with cooling coconut milk, musky fish sauce with sharp lime. It's an exciting cuisine that dances on your taste buds.

- 4 tablespoons dried mint
- 2 tablespoons fresh lime zest
- 4 teaspoons ground white pepper
- 2 teaspoons ground black pepper
- 2 teaspoons fresh lemongrass, minced
- ¼ teaspoon ground cumin
- ½ teaspoon cayenne powder
- 1 tablespoon dried cilantro
- 1 tablespoon unsweetened shredded coconut

Mix together all the ingredients. Store in the freezer in an airtight container.

SPANISH SPICE BLEND

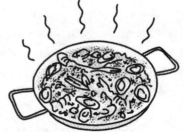

Yield: 1 cup

I like to use this blend with seafood and chicken as they do with paella and seafood stews in Spain. It works well with quinoa and brown rice as well. This blend is so flavorful, you might want to use it in a dip.

Saffron, which looks like pieces of thin red-orange thread, is often used in Spanish cuisine. Its pungent flavor is difficult to describe—some say it is floral, and others think it is like honey. Saffron turns food bright yellow, which significantly contributes to the visual appeal of food. Saffron is the most expensive spice in the world. To make a pound of saffron, more than two hundred thousand stigmas from crocus flowers must be harvested by hand. Because it's so pricey, even in small quantities, I have made saffron an optional ingredient in this blend.

6 tablespoons smoked paprika

3 tablespoons sweet paprika

I tablespoon chili powder

3 tablespoons dried cilantro

2 tablespoons onion powder

I tablespoon ground cumin

I tablespoon fresh lemon zest

1½ teaspoons ground black pepper

Pinch of saffron (optional)

Mix together all the ingredients. Store in the freezer in an airtight container.

MOROCCAN SPICE BLEND

Yield: ⅓ cup

The word *Morocco* evokes an exotic, mysterious place. Couscous and beef and chicken tagines are well known dishes from Moroccan cuisine. The layered quality of this blend is memorable as it mixes sweet, pungent, and hot flavors. It pairs well with seafood, lamb, poultry, beef, veggies, beans, and lentils.

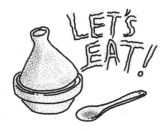

2 tablespoons ground cumin

I tablespoon paprika

I tablespoon ground coriander

I teaspoon freshly ground black pepper

I teaspoon ground cinnamon

I teaspoon ground allspice

¼ teaspoon ground cloves

⅛ teaspoon cayenne pepper, or to taste

Mix together all the ingredients in an airtight container and store in a cool, dry place away from heat and light.

MEDITERRANEAN SPICE BLEND

Yield: about 6 tablespoons

You would have to be living in a cave if you weren't aware of the health benefits of Mediterranean cuisine. This blend will take you to a *taverna* near the port on a Greek island, where the fishermen come with their catch.

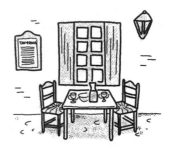

- 1 tablespoon garlic powder
- 1 tablespoon onion powder
- 1 tablespoon dried parsley
- 2 teaspoons dried oregano
- 2 teaspoons fine sea salt

- 1 teaspoon freshly ground black pepper
- 1 teaspoon dried thyme
- 1 teaspoon fresh lemon zest
- ½ teaspoon ground cinnamon

Mix together all the ingredients. Store in the freezer in an airtight container.

FALAFEL SPICE BLEND

Yield: about 3 tablespoons

Middle Eastern food has been growing in popularity all over the country. Hummus, baba ghanoush, tabbouleh, chicken, lamb and beef shawarma, tzatziki, and lamb gyros are just a few examples of the extraordinary food from the Middle East. In some cities, Middle Eastern vendors and restaurants are on every corner. This is great party food!

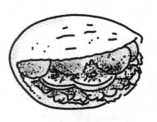

- 2 teaspoons smoked paprika
- 2 teaspoons ground cumin
- 1 teaspoon ground black pepper
- 1 teaspoon ground coriander

- ½ teaspoon ground cinnamon
- ½ teaspoon ground nutmeg
- ¼ teaspoon ground cardamom
- ¼ teaspoon ground cloves

Mix together all the ingredients in an airtight container and store in a cool, dry place away from heat and light.

How Much to Use

For any dish that serves four to six people, use ½ teaspoon of ground spice or dried herbs. For chopped fresh herbs, use 1½ teaspoons. Since oils are concentrated in the drying process of herbs and spices, it takes about a third the quantity of dried herbs as fresh.

In general, add ground or chopped spices and herbs around the midway point or toward the end of the cooking process so their flavors stay strong.

THE SWISS ARMY KNIFE OF SPICE BLENDS

I have put together these at-a-glance charts to give you some ideas of what type of food might pair well with each blend. You can use them to mix and match flavor ideas, and of course get creative on your own with any combination you'd like to try!

Foundational

	Chicken	*Beef*	*Pork*	*Lamb*	*Fish*	*Shellfish*	*Veggies*
Salt-Free "Better than Salt" Blend	✔	✔	✔	✔	✔	✔	✔
Savory Soup Blend	✔	✔	✔	✔	✔	✔	✔
Poultry Spice Blend	✔		✔		✔		✔
Veggies Never Tasted Like This Blend							✔

United States of Flavors

	Chicken	Beef	Pork	Lamb	Fish	Shellfish	Veggies
N'awlins Spiced Pecan Crust Blend	✔			✔	✔		
Nuts 4 Almonds Coconut Crust Blend	✔	✔	✔	✔	✔	✔	✔
Little Italy Blend	✔	✔	✔		✔	✔	✔
Sour Dill Pickle Blend	✔				✔	✔	✔
Granddad's BBQ Blend	✔	✔	✔		✔	✔	
Chesapeake Bay Crab and Seafood Blend	✔				✔	✔	✔
Tex-Mex Chili Blend	✔	✔					✔
Blackened Spice Blend	✔	✔			✔		
Sunshine Citrus Blend	✔					✔	✔
Bayou Cajun Blend	✔	✔			✔	✔	✔

Global

	Chicken	Beef	Pork	Lamb	Fish	Shellfish	Veggies
Fiesta Spice Blend	✔	✔			✔	✔	✔
Zesty Parmesan Blend	✔						✔
Jamaican Me Crazy Jerk Spice Blend	✔		✔		✔	✔	

	1	2	3	4	5	6	7	8
Japanese-Inspired Blend						✔	✔	✔
Indian Masala Spice Blend	✔	✔	✔			✔	✔	✔
Year of the Dragon Chinese Marinade	✔	✔		✔		✔		✔
Thai Spice Blend	✔	✔	✔			✔	✔	✔
Spanish Spice Blend	✔					✔	✔	✔
Moroccan Spice Blend	✔	✔		✔				✔
Mediterranean Spice Blend	✔			✔		✔	✔	✔
Falafel Spice Blend	✔	✔		✔				✔

SPICE COMPATIBILITY

Some spices simply do not go together. For whatever reason, their flavors don't meld when combined, or they can actually clash. As you begin to have fun with spices in your cooking and want to create your own combinations, you might be baffled about which spices go well together. The chart that follows gives you a quick reference to what spices blend together well and what foods are compatible with a specific spice. As you gain more confidence, you will come up with different creative blends. Experiment! The possibilities are countless.

If you are feeling insecure about experimenting, think about salt and pepper. You know when you have been heavy-handed with either of these seasonings. The same is true for spices and herbs. Start with modest measurements and add spices and herbs to taste. Remember: Dried spices and powders are more intense than fresh herbs. The rule of thumb is that 1 tablespoon fresh herbs equals 1 teaspoon dried—that's a 3:1 ratio. When you're trying a new combination, though, start off lightly and taste your way up to the perfect flavor.

Spice	Blends With	Good With
Allspice	Cardamom, cinnamon, ginger, nutmeg	Apples, beets, cabbage, nuts, onions, pears, poultry, root vegetables, seafood
Basil	Garlic, parsley, lemongrass, chili, oregano, rosemary, coriander, mint, thyme	Tomato, olive oil, onion, chicken, pasta, eggs, zucchini, strawberries, spinach, eggplant, leafy vegetables, mushrooms, olives, peaches, poultry, raspberries, seafood
Cayenne/chile	Cilantro, cinnamon, cumin, basil, garlic, ginger, oregano	Bananas, beans, grains, cheese, citrus, chocolate, corn, beef, potatoes, poultry, seafood, tropical fruits
Cinnamon	Allspice, cardamom, chiles, clove, curry, ginger, nutmeg	Apples, bananas, beans, chocolate, coffee, cranberry, dates, game meats, grains, squash, tea
Coriander	Cilantro, cumin, mint, parsley	Bananas, beans, cured meats, curry, game meats, poultry, root vegetables, seafood, tomatoes
Cumin	Cilantro, garlic, mint, parsley	Avocados, beans, beef, citrus, cucumber, grains, mango, onion, poultry, sausages, seafood, tomatoes
Dill	Aniseed, caraway, chives, fennel, mint, oregano, parsley, tarragon	Beets, blue cheese, cabbage, carrots, chicken soup, cucumbers, eggs, potatoes, seafood, tomatoes, veal
Garlic	Basil, chile, coriander, dill, ginger, marjoram, oregano, parsley, rosemary, sage, thyme, turmeric	Beans, beef, chicken, lamb, mushrooms, onions, pasta, pork, potatoes, seafood, spinach
Ginger	Allspice, aniseed, chiles, chives, cinnamon, cloves, coriander, cumin, fennel, garlic, nutmeg, pepper	Asparagus, bananas, carrots, chocolate, citrus, coconut, cranberry, curry, dates, onions, pears, poultry, raisins, root vegetables, seafood, tea, tropical fruits

Nutmeg	Allspice, cinnamon, clove, cumin, ginger	Asparagus, blue cheese, cabbage, carrots, cheese, cranberries, coffee, eggs, green beans, pasta, peaches, pumpkin, potato
Oregano	Basil, cinnamon, cumin, fennel, garlic, parsley, thyme	Artichokes, beans, beef, blue cheese, eggplant, mushrooms, nuts, pasta, poultry, seafood, squash, tomatoes, veal
Paprika	Allspice, basil, caraway, cardamom, chile, cinnamon, cloves, coriander, cumin, fennel, garlic, ginger, oregano, parsley, rosemary, sage, thyme, turmeric	Veal, pork, chicken, beef, eggs, sauces
Parsley	Basil, bay leaf, chervil, chives, dill, garlic, oregano, rosemary, thyme	Artichokes, asparagus, beets, beef, game meats, grains, mushrooms, onions, pasta, potatoes, poultry, sea food, tomatoes
Rosemary	Basil, garlic, fennel, oregano, parsley, sage, thyme	Apples, asparagus, beans, beef, blue cheese, citrus, cranberry, game meats, grains, mushrooms, nuts, onion, potatoes, poultry, seafood, tomatoes
Sage	Garlic, parsley, rosemary, thyme	Anchovy, capers, cranberry, beef, game meats, green beans, mushrooms, nuts, pasta, plums, poultry, seafood, veal
Thyme	Basil, bay leaf, chervil, dill, mint, oregano, parsley, sage	Artichoke, bananas, beans, carrots, citrus, cranberry, dates, mushrooms, nuts, onion, potatoes, poultry, seafood, tomatoes
Turmeric	Allspice, cardamom, chile, fennel, garlic, ginger, lemongrass, paprika, parsley	Chicken, vegetables, seafood, curries, tagines, soup, roasted vegetables, leafy greens

LET'S LOOK AT IT ANOTHER WAY: PAIRING VEGETABLES AND FRUIT WITH HERBS

Sometimes, you can look at a head of broccoli or some green beans that you are planning to steam and just not know what spices and herbs to use to layer on the flavor. The lists that follow will give you the information you need to make pairing spices and herbs with vegetables a snap. I have listed the information by vegetable. I want to make it as easy as possible for you to enhance the flavor of vegetables and fruits, because one of your primary aims in changing the way you eat is to increase your consumption of plant foods. You will be surprised at some of the fruit pairings. You may think that there is nothing as good as fresh berries or peaches, but wait until you try them with fresh basil or mint. Delicious!

Vegetables

Artichokes: bay leaf, parsley, oregano, red pepper flakes, thyme

Asparagus: chervil, chives, curry, dill, garlic, lemon, mustard, onion, sesame seeds, tarragon

Beets: allspice, basil, caraway, coriander, dill, fennel seeds, ginger, horseradish, mint, star anise, tarragon

Broccoli: caraway, curry, dill, ginger, mint, oregano, red pepper flakes, savory, turmeric

Brussels sprouts: basil, caraway, dill, parsley, nutmeg, paprika

Cabbage: caraway seeds, celery seeds, coriander, curry, dill, fennel seeds, ginger, mint, savory, tarragon, thyme

Carrots: allspice, basil, bay leaf, caraway seeds, chervil, cinnamon, cloves, coriander, fennel greens, ginger, mace, mint, parsley, sage, star anise, tarragon, thyme

Cauliflower: basil, caraway seeds, chives, coriander, curry, dill, fennel seeds, paprika, sage, thyme, turmeric

Celery: basil, chervil, curry, dill, paprika, parsley

Corn: basil, chives, cilantro, dill seeds, oregano, parsley, rosemary, thyme

Cucumber: allspice, basil, coriander, dill, mint, mustard, parsley, tarragon

Eggplant: basil, cumin, curry, marjoram, oregano, parsley, red pepper flakes, rosemary, savory, thyme

Fennel bulb: basil, caraway seeds, coriander, nutmeg, parsley, paprika, rosemary, thyme

Green beans: basil, chives, dill, onion, oregano, rosemary, savory

Kale: allspice, caraway, chile, coriander, dill, marjoram, mustard, nutmeg, tarragon, thyme

Leeks: caraway, dill, mustard, paprika, nutmeg

Lettuce: neutral, can be mixed with any spice or herb

Mushrooms: marjoram, nutmeg, parsley, oregano, sage, tarragon, and thyme

Onions: aniseed, basil, bay leaf, caraway seeds, cloves, curry, mustard seeds, nutmeg, oregano, paprika, parsley, thyme

Peas: chervil, chives, curry, dill, mint, nutmeg, parsley, rosemary, tarragon, thyme, turmeric

Peppers: basil, curry, ginger, mustard, oregano, paprika, parsley, rosemary, thyme

Potatoes: caraway seeds, chervil, chives, dill, dill seeds, mace, marjoram, paprika, parsley, rosemary, sage, thyme, turmeric

Pumpkin: celery leaves, chives, curry, ginger, onions, sage, thyme

Radishes: basil, chives, dill, mint, parsley

Red cabbage: basil, bay leaf, caraway, cloves, ginger, nutmeg, onions, thyme

Spinach: allspice, basil, chives, dill, nutmeg, sesame seeds, thyme

Squash, summer: basil, chives, coriander, dill, marjoram, onions, oregano

Squash, winter: celery leaves, coriander, mace, marjoram, onions, parsley, sage

Sweet potatoes: allspice, cardamom, chile, cinnamon, cloves, ginger, nutmeg, sage, thyme

Swiss Chard: allspice, marjoram, nutmeg, paprika, parsley, savory

Tomatoes: allspice, basil, cilantro, cumin, curry, dill, fennel seeds, garlic, oregano, parsley, paprika, red pepper flakes, rosemary, tarragon, thyme

Fruit

Apricots: cardamom, dill, ginger, lime zest, vanilla

Apples: cardamom, cilantro, cinnamon, cloves, ginger, mint, nutmeg

Bananas: cardamom, cilantro, cinnamon, cloves, coriander, ginger, parsley, thyme

Berries: aniseed, basil, cardamom, cinnamon, cloves, coriander, ginger, mace, mint, nutmeg, pepper, star anise

Blackberries: cinnamon, ginger, mint, pink peppercorns

Blueberries: ginger, lemon grass, lemon zest, lime zest, orange zest

Cantaloupe: basil, cilantro, cinnamon, ginger, lemongrass, mint, nutmeg, pepper, vanilla

Cherries: basil, mint, lemon zest, orange zest, thyme, vanilla

Dates: cinnamon, ginger, orange zest, vanilla

Figs: aniseeed, cardamom, fennel seed, ginger, mace, mint, rosemary, thyme

Grapes: basil, cardamom, cinnamon, cloves, garlic powder, ground ginger, mint, nutmeg, parsley, rosemary, star anise, thyme, vanilla

Grapefruit: basil, cardamom, cinnamon, cloves, fresh ginger, mint, nutmeg, parsley, rosemary, tarragon

Guava: basil, ginger, mint, poppy seed

Honeydew melon: cilantro, mint, thyme

Lemon: black pepper, cinnamon, cumin, dill, ginger, red pepper flakes, vanilla

Lime: basil, cilantro, lemongrass

Mangoes: cayenne, chili powder, cilantro, peppermint

Oranges: cardamom, fennel seed, mint, thyme

Peaches: basil, cloves, mint, nutmeg, thyme

Pears: bay leaf, cardamom, cilantro, cinnamon, mint, pepper, star anise, thyme

Pineapple: cloves, ginger, lemongrass, mint, rosemary

Plums: basil, cinnamon, cloves, nutmeg, star anise

Pumpkin: allspice, black sesame seeds, cardamom, cinnamon, clove, ginger, nutmeg, sage, thyme, vanilla, honey

Raspberries: chive, cinnamon, mint, pink peppercorn, star anise

Rhubarb: cinnamon, ginger, pepper, vanilla

Strawberries: allspice, basil, balsamic vinegar, cocoa powder, mint, nutmeg

Summer melons: cilantro, mint, parsley, thyme

CREATING YOUR OWN SPICE BLENDS

The twenty-five spice blends in this chapter cover a lot of flavor territory. As you get more experienced and identify the flavors you like the most, you might want to tweak the spice blends I have provided by changing the proportion of the ingredients. After a time, you might want to craft your own blends to produce unique tastes and aromas that appeal to you. As your taste buds become more sensitized, you will appreciate the subtle flavors contributing to the blend.

Balance is the key to making a spice blend that works. In chapter 2, you learned about how spices are categorized: sweet, pungent, tangy, hot, and amalgamating. Here are some guidelines:

- Sweet spices can balance the flavor of more powerful spices.
- Since pungent spices are strong, you have to use them sparingly.
- Tangy spices are astringent and add another important dimension.
- Use hot spices in very small amounts.
- Amalgamating spices tie other spices together.
- If you need to make a correction, sweet paprika is an amalgamating spice you can use to bring the blend back into balance.

The Spice and Herb Bible, which is a valuable resource, gives approximate proportions of the types of spices in a blend. As you create a blend, remember that you want to satisfy all your taste buds so that you hit that bliss point. A balanced blend of dried ingredients should contain:

- 2 percent hot spices
- 4 percent pungent spices/herbs
- 12 percent tangy spices/strong herbs
- 22 percent sweet spices/medium herbs
- 60 percent amalgamating spices/mild herbs

Hot Spices (2 percent): chile, horseradish, mustard, pepper

Pungent Spices and Herbs (4 percent): bay leaf, caraway, cardamom, celery seed, cloves, cumin, dill seed, fenugreek seed, garlic, ginger, mace, oregano, rosemary, sage, savory, star anise, thyme

Tangy Spices and Strong Herbs (12 percent): basil, cilantro, dill, fenugreek, lemongrass, marjoram, mint, tarragon

Sweet Spices and Medium Herbs (22 percent): allspice, aniseed, cinnamon, chives, nutmeg

Amalgamating Spices and Mild Herbs (60 percent): chervil, coriander seed, fennel seed, filé powder, paprika, parsley, poppy seed, sesame seed, turmeric

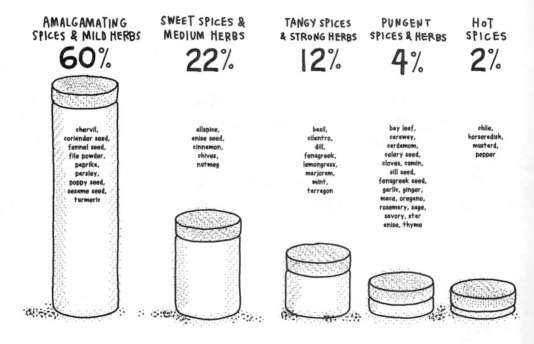

12

LIFETIME STRATEGIES

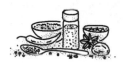

Now you know what you should be eating to achieve your ideal weight and to be as healthy as you can be. You have been following the meals plans for the first thirty days of Phase 1 of the Spice Diet, as well as preparing the recipes I've created. You've seen how powerhouse flavor reduces your cravings. Your cooking skills have improved, and you should be feeling more at ease in the kitchen. In fact, you should be proud of the excellent food you make yourself. You will find yourself reaching for spices and spice blends automatically now. When you enjoy making your own meals and snacks, being mindful about what you eat is built into the process of planning, shopping for, and preparing your food. Your food choices expand when you graduate to Phase 2. You are eating the way you need to in order to maintain your weight loss. You have the logistics down and have formed some good habits. You are on your way to a lifetime of healthy eating.

As you are making changes to your eating and adding movement to your life, don't expect to be perfect all the time. The key is not to let one meal or one day's eating that is off the charts lead you totally off course. There will be relapses—it happens to everyone. Some people build in an "anything goes" meal or day into their eating plan. They allow themselves to eat whatever they want for a meal or even an entire day on a regular basis.

When I go a little crazy, which, I have to confess, I allow myself to do every now and then, I end up not feeling good. I have become so used to eating well that eating the food I used to crave isn't as satisfying and has consequences. The taste of junk food just doesn't hold up to the flavor of fresh, whole food seasoned with natural herbs and spices. My body has become accustomed to nutrient-dense food that doesn't put me on the blood sugar roller coaster. I've worked so hard to get where I am now with my weight that a long detour is the last thing I want to do. Even so, there are times when the temptation of going off plan is especially strong.

I'm sure your determination will be challenged on many occasions that are difficult for anyone. Eating out, finding yourself with your children at a fast-food restaurant or simply not being able to resist the drive-thru, getting through parties and celebrations without losing control, not to mention the entire holiday season, and traveling for business or vacation—these situations can create havoc with your normal eating routine. I have given a good deal of thought—and practice—to dealing with these potential pitfalls without succumbing to my old behaviors. This chapter will give you some tried-and-true strategies that get me through times that could easily trip me up.

EATING OUT WITHOUT BLOWING ALL YOUR GOOD WORK

According to a 2013 survey conducted by Living Social, Americans have become a nation that eats out four or five times a week. Eating out is one of our favorite pastimes. Aside from convenience, it's fun to go out with friends or to treat the family to a good meal at a restaurant. From the menu choices to the breadbasket, from the size of the portions to the dessert cart, the problem with eating out is that it is easy to give in to temptation and eat too much of the wrong things.

Just as you have learned to be prepared for when you eat at home, it is important to have a plan when you go to a restaurant. To make sure you don't throw all caution to the wind when you go out to dinner, here are some strategies for sticking with the plan. I have compiled these strategies based on my own experience as well as tips from family, friends, and people with whom I have worked.

The Dining-Out Dozen

1. **Look over the menu before you go.** Banish the thought of a buffet restaurant from your mind and plans. Eating at an "all you can

eat" buffet is an invitation to diet disaster. If you have never been to the restaurant you choose, check out the menu ahead of time. Decide what you want to order before you leave your house to avoid making snap decisions that you might regret later. Foods described as fried, crispy, panfried, crunchy, or sautéed can be a mother lode of fat and calories. You want to choose food that has been grilled, roasted, poached, or steamed. If you decide you must order that eggplant Parmesan or those cold sesame noodles, you can eat very carefully earlier in the day to keep your caloric intake from soaring. Remember: you don't have to eat the whole portion. After the meal, take a menu home with you so you have it on hand if you decide to order in at a later date.

2. **Make reservations if you are going to a busy place.** Waiting for a table only gives you time to get hungry. If you have to wait, you might order drinks at the bar or nibble on the snacks offered there. Ask for or find a quiet table away from the kitchen. You can lose track of how much you are eating when there are too many distractions. If there is too much bustle, you can devour your food quickly. When seated near the kitchen, you have a perfect view of all the dishes as they pass by on their way to be served. That parade of decadent food can weaken your resolve about what you had planned to order.

3. **Going to a restaurant hungry is asking for trouble.** Make sure to have a healthy snack an hour before you are set to leave so that you don't arrive at the restaurant famished. If you want more room to indulge when you are out, I suggest that you eat smaller meals and reduce your caloric intake during the day.

4. **Follow the one-drink rule.** Alcohol can stimulate your appetite and cause the calories to pile up. If you start with a drink on an empty stomach, your self-control could dissolve. Drink water, unsweetened iced tea, or a spicy Virgin Mary before the food arrives. During the meal, treat yourself to glass of wine if you would like, but also drink plenty of water.

5. **Say "no" to the breadbasket.** Have you ever noticed that when you sit down at a restaurant, complimentary treats quickly materialize? Bread, rolls, focaccia with butter or olive oil, dips and

crackers, tortilla chips, papadums, fried noodles, or marinated
olives arrive when you are most vulnerable. If others at the table
agree, send the server away with the treats, so you won't be
tempted to eat high-calorie starters mindlessly. Drink a big glass of
ice water if your friends or family want to indulge.

6. **Be the first to order.** Because you have studied the menu and
   made your selections, you can order while everyone else decides
   what to eat. You don't want to be influenced by what everyone else
   is having.

7. **Have it your way.** Don't be shy about making special requests.
   Most restaurants will accommodate you if you ask for food to be
   prepared as you would like. Chefs know that customers are more
   health conscious than ever. You can ask if the chef will steam,
   poach, broil, grill, or bake a dish rather than fry it. You might
   request that the chef substitute extra-virgin olive oil instead of
   butter, or leave the cheese out of the salad. You can usually make
   healthy substitutions, such as steamed veggies, a salad, a baked
   potato, or sweet potatoes instead of French fries or mashed potatoes. Assume that you have some control over how your food is
   prepared.

8. **Always have dressings and sauces on the side.** Restaurants tend
   to smother salad with too much dressing and oversauce many
   dishes, which adds many calories to your meal. One way to cut
   back on those calories is to have the dressing or sauce served on
   the side. By dipping the tines of your fork into the dressing or
   sauce before you take a bite of the food, you will get the flavor as
   you minimize your calorie consumption.

9. **Order appetizers and/or side dishes as a main course.** The
   beauty of this strategy is that portion control is not an issue. A
   salad and an appetizer can be a terrific meal. Seafood, grilled vegetables, and broth-based soups are excellent choices. Stay away from
   creamy, fried, and cheesy choices and anything in a pastry crust.

10. **Just because it's a salad doesn't mean it's calorie-free.** Stay
    away from tuna, chicken, potato, coleslaw, and macaroni salads,
    which are often full of sugar and mayonnaise. Go for vegetables,
    fresh greens, and beans without the killer add-ons like cheese,

bacon, croutons, sweetened nuts, and dried fruit. Beware of the chicken Caesar salad, which can be high in fat and calories. Use fresh lemon or vinaigrette for dressings. Remember to control the amount of dressing used by ordering it on the side.

11. **You don't have to eat everything on your plate.** So many restaurants serve jumbo portions. There is no need to eat until you can't take another bite just because it is in front of you. If you eat slowly, you can stop when you feel satisfied. It takes twenty minutes for your body to register that you are full. If you know the restaurant serves big portions in advance, you can share the dish with someone else or order a half portion. Don't be shy about asking for a doggie bag. Having leftovers for another meal is a bonus!

12. **Pass on dessert.** If you want to eat something sweet at the end of the meal, order fresh fruit. Berries are a good choice. If your sweet tooth is making dessert too difficult to resist, share a luscious dessert or order a couple of desserts for the table. Try to have only three or four bites, and really enjoy them. If the pastry chef is a genius or is known for her pecan pie, order it. You don't have to eat all of it. The first three or four bites of anything are always the best. Stop after that. It's a question of diminishing returns after those initial tastes. Offer what is left on your plate to your friends and family or ask your server to take the plate away if there are no takers. My advice is to not take dessert leftovers home. I still have visions of myself waking up in the middle of the night with the dessert calling me from the refrigerator. I can do without those wee-hour struggles with myself. If you make a conscious decision to indulge in a sinfully rich dessert, enjoy it, but be very careful of what you eat for the next few days.

The Dining-Out Dozen is a guide to enjoying restaurant meals without going over the top and losing your focus on healthy eating. Because ethnic and fast-food restaurants can pose particular challenges to maintaining your commitment to eating healthy, following are some suggestions for dealing with those situations.

Healthy Eating in the Melting Pot

Our country is composed of people of so many nationalities that it is no wonder that a variety of ethnic food is so popular. With every wave of immigrants, we have welcomed the new flavors that their cuisines bring to us. You can find restaurants with cuisine from all over the world in big cities and small towns. Americans seem more and more open to trying new flavors. The choices are abundant. Everyone seems to go out for or order takeout from popular global food, including Chinese, Mexican, Italian, Japanese, Greek, French, Thai, Spanish, and Indian, which have become staples in the diets of many Americans. In the spice blends in chapter 11, I have tried to capture many of these flavor profiles so you can reproduce them at home. But if you are going to eat out, here is how best to do it. When you order from an ethnic menu, you have to be careful to avoid choosing that cuisine's equivalent of a double cheeseburger and fries. Let's take a look at what foods from the cuisines of these countries are compatible with the way you want to eat. The cuisines are listed in order of their popularity in the United States, according to food research from Technomic for *Parade* magazine.

Chinese

If you are not careful about your choices, you can end up consuming more calories, fat, and sodium than is good for you. When it comes to Chinese food, egg rolls and sesame noodles top the list of American favorites. Neither is an excellent choice. Chinese food is a sophisticated cuisine that has so much to offer that will work with your new way of eating.

Do:

- Use chopsticks, which will force you to eat more slowly.
- Ask for your food to be prepared without MSG, a flavor enhancer that can bring on side effects such as headaches, flushing, tingling in the mouth, and dizziness. If an ingredient can cause this sort of reaction, it is worth avoiding.
- Start with hot-and-sour or egg drop soup.
- Try vegetables for appetizers—for example, lettuce wraps like chicken *soong* or vegetable spring rolls.
- Order stir-fries made with little or no oil and lots of vegetables.

- Going for anything steamed is a good choice. Dumplings, vegetables, seafood, a whole fish, chicken, and meat taste great when steamed.
- Chinese sauces can be loaded with salt, sugar, and fat. You can order sauce on the side or ask if the dish can be made with half the sauce. Ask for low-sodium soy sauce.
- Request brown rice if it is available.

DON'T:

- Order anything fried. Wontons, shrimp toast, fried rice, and egg rolls, Kung Pao chicken, General Tso's chicken, sesame chicken, ginger beef, and sweet-and-sour pork all fall into that category.
- Have fatty spareribs.
- Order Peking duck. Although most of the fat is drained off in preparation, the crispy skin—the best part of the dish as far as I'm concerned—is not good for your waistline.
- Eat "Mandarin pancakes" or wraps. Eat your moo shu vegetables, pork, or chicken without the flour pancakes.

Mexican

Believe me, I know that Mexican food can be a caloric disaster. Eating high-fat meats, sour cream, cheese, refried beans, and deep-fried combo plates can really pack on the pounds. But many Mexican dishes are healthier and derive strong flavors from garlic, lime and citrus juice, oregano, and chile. There are plenty of dishes you can eat and stay on plan. I've had to grapple with Mexican menus for a long time and have come up with a long list of recommendations.

DO:

- Forget about beer, and save the margarita—without salt—until the food arrives, if you must.
- Order ceviche as an appetizer. Protein-rich ceviche is made from fresh raw fish or scallops that have been marinated with lime juice.
- Order corn tortillas, which are lower in fat and calories than flour tortillas.
- Choose grilled fish, shrimp, and chicken.
- Consider salads without a taco shell or cheese, and vegetable stews.

- Order fajitas made with shrimp, chicken, or beef. You don't have to eat the soft tacos. Ask the waitperson to hold back on the sour cream and cheese. Use salsa or a little guacamole.
- Look for Veracruz sauce, which is made from tomatoes, onions, and chiles.
- Try *pico de gallo*, a salsa made from chopped tomato, onion, cilantro, fresh hot peppers, salt, and lime juice, as a salad dressing or a condiment on everything. Use *salsa verde* or green sauce the same way. This tart, vibrant sauce is made from tomatillos, small tomato-like fruits that grow in a papery husk.
- Eat chicken enchiladas without the cheese. Just eat the filling and not the baked corn tortilla.
- Try the fish tacos without the taco shell.
- Ask if the rice and beans are cooked in lard. If so, they are not for you. Black beans and rice might be a better choice.
- Order a tostada without the cheese. Consider the crispy flat taco—that the beans, meat, and salsa are piled on a plate.
- Fall in love with mole sauce. It is a blend of nuts, seeds, spices, a number of chile peppers, and, last but not least, Mexican chocolate. Talk about depth of flavor! It's great on chicken.

DON'T:

- Dive into the basket of tortilla chips. Use the guacamole or salsa that comes with the chips as a sauce.
- Even think about eating nachos.
- Order deep-fried dishes like *sopapillas*, *chimichangas*, and *flautas*.
- Pile on the cheese and sour cream. Use guacamole as a sauce instead.
- Order anything in a *suiza* sauce, which is made from cheese and often condensed milk.
- Eat refried beans.

Italian

Italian food has been popular for so long that it doesn't seem ethnic anymore. Italy is the home of the Mediterranean diet—with its core ingredients of tomatoes, olive oil, garlic, basil, oregano, and parsley. Tons of gooey melted cheese is not part of traditional Italian cooking—that's an Italian American add-on. A small amount of grated hard cheese, such as Pecorino Romano or Parmigiano Reggiano, is the flavor boost of choice for classic Italian cooking. For the healthiest meal, you have to eat like an Italian. Gigantic portions of pasta smothered in cheese, served as a main course here in the United States, would feed a family of six in Italy. Portion control is the key to enjoying whole wheat pasta without carbo loading.

Do:

- Skip the breadbasket, even the breadsticks, and especially the focaccia. Did you know that a piece of focaccia could have double the calories of a piece of bread?
- Sample Italian soups. Those that combine escarole, beans, and sausage are like a stew—very filling and tasty. Italian wedding soup, minestrone, and cioppino, which is a seafood-broth-based soup, are a great way to start a meal. In fact, soup with a side salad can *be* the meal.
- Make a meal from antipasti. There are so many wonderful foods to choose from: olives, marinated and grilled vegetables, caponata, artichokes, asparagus, grilled calamari, giant fava beans, garbanzo beans, also known as chickpeas, and cannellini bean salads, shrimp cocktail, even very thinly sliced dried meats like prosciutto, bresaola, and mortadella.
- A steamed artichoke is a great way to start a meal—it keeps you busy as you pluck leaf after leaf. Use lemon instead of butter for a dipping sauce.
- Order hollow pastas like orecchiette and ziti, because your portion will look larger.
- Order whole wheat pasta.
- Look for things in prepared with marinara, fra Diavolo, puttanesca, piccata, or with marsala sauce.
- Order pasta with clam sauce or pasta primavera with fresh vegetables. You can concentrate on the clams or vegetables and leave most of the pasta behind.
- Eat only half your pasta order. Take the rest home.
- Enjoy terrific Italian salads such as tricolore or arugula. Make certain the salad isn't loaded with cheese. As always, ask for dressing on the side so you are in control of how much you use.

- Opt for grilled or roasted fish prepared with garlic, lemon, and olive oil or shellfish cooked in a broth for your main course. The same with simple roasted chicken or chicken marsala. Make sure the fish or chicken is not breaded.
- A rich, fragrant espresso with biscotti is a perfect dessert.

Don't:

- Order anything stuffed, for example, mushrooms, clams, artichokes, or pasta shells.
- Eat anything breaded or deep-fried like chicken Milanese, even though it has a salad on top.
- Indulge in a Caesar salad. The croutons, cheese, and rich dressing do not make for a caloric bargain.
- Eat anything in creamy Alfredo sauce.
- Go for gooey lasagna, manicotti, or deep-dish pepperoni pizza.
- Consider eggplant a healthy vegetable. It acts like a sponge to soak up all the oil in a dish.

Japanese

Japanese food has become the dieter's special. Eating clean is easier to do with this cuisine. Most Japanese food is prepared in a healthy way, either steamed, boiled, or raw. The mainstays of the cuisine are extremely healthy: omega 3-rich seafood, veggies like bok choy that are packed with calcium, vitamin- and mineral-rich seaweed and mushrooms, and whole soy foods. Here are some tips on healthy eating at Japanese restaurants:

Do:

- Use chopsticks to slow you down.
- Leave some sauce at the bottom of the bowl, because Japanese sauces tend to be very salty.
- Request low-sodium soy sauce.
- Ask for sauce on the side.
- Order a cucumber, seaweed, or house salad with ginger dressing on the side as a starter.
- Include cold spinach with sesame and steamed vegetable gyoza, or dumplings, in your list of starter options.

- Season your food with wasabi, chile sauce, or ginger.
- Order brown rice if it is available.
- Order vegetable "sushi" rolls or classic rolls with simple ingredients.
- Choose sashimi over sushi.
- Go with salmon over tuna, because mercury levels are high in tuna.
- Try chicken or salmon teriyaki.
- Eat *sukiyaki*, a hot-pot dish, usually cooked at the table in a cast-iron skillet filled with broth. It typically contains thinly sliced beef, cubes of tofu, and a variety of fresh vegetables. Use the dipping sauces sparingly.
- Give soba noodles a try. They are made of buckwheat.

Don't:

- Drink sake, which is liquid rice. A 6-ounce glass of sake has about 230 calories compared to 150 calories for the same size serving of wine.
- Order tempura, which is fried.
- Eat udon noodles made from wheat.

Greek

Greek cuisine is another form of a Mediterranean diet. Dark, leafy vegetables, high-fiber beans, fresh fruit, olives, nuts, lentils, grains, olive oil, and lots of fish are all health promoting. Studies have shown that people lose more weight and feel more satisfied on a Mediterranean diet, which is rich in healthy fats, than on a low-fat diet.

Do:

- Enjoy Greek salad, but be mindful of the feta cheese. Although feta is lower in fat than other cheeses, it is salty and adds calories. It's a good idea to push half the feta cheese aside.
- Serve yourself spreads such as hummus and tzatziki directly onto your plate. That way you can keep track of how much you are eating, preferably no more than 2 tablespoons, and say no to the pita bread.
- Order grilled fish and spinach or other greens sautéed with olive oil and garlic.

- Have roast or grilled chicken, which the Greeks season beautifully.
- Enjoy chicken kebabs.
- Have a lamb souvlaki platter with grilled vegetables and tzatziki rather than a lamb gyro.
- Skip the rice and pita.
- Enjoy nonfat Greek yogurt and fresh fruit for dessert.

Don't:

- Eat moussaka, the Greek version of lasagna, made with eggplant and a rich, creamy topping. A serving is a calorie bomb.
- Order anything with phyllo pastry, such as spanakopita. This spinach pie can be as caloric and fat laden as a bacon cheeseburger.
- Be seduced by Greek desserts like baklava, which are swimming in butter and honey with nuts on top.

French

I studied at the famed Cordon Bleu in Paris and worked at the five-star Ritz Hotel there. All that cream, butter, rich sauce, and extraordinary cheese, not to mention remarkable pastries, tarts, and cake, is fabulous and luxurious. French women stay so chicly thin by limiting the size of their portions drastically. The truth is, a few bites can be enough. Savor each mouthful of this splendid cuisine. In addition to portion control, ordering simply is the best way to go.

Do:

- Choose broth-based soups, like bouillabaisse, a traditional fish stew, or *soupe au pistou*, a vegetable soup made with pesto.
- Enjoy how the French do wonders with leeks and endives.
- Order *coquilles St-Jacques*, as scallops are called, and mussels.
- Try a *salade Niçoise*, made with lettuce, green beans, olives, and fresh tuna.
- Fall back on an omelet when you are in doubt. French omelets are superb!
- Have a *salade chèvre chaud* for lunch. It is a small green salad with a thin round of baked chèvre (goat cheese) on top. Delicious!
- Stick to light vinaigrette dressings.

- Try beef bourguignonne, a spectacular beef stew made with red wine, but watch the size of your portion—no more than three ounces of beef, which is the size of a deck of cards or the palm of your hand.
- Sample *choucroute garnie*, a sauerkraut, meat, and boiled potato dish from Alsace—don't have a whole serving.
- Splurge on dessert. French baking is extraordinary. The confections created by pastry chefs are mind-boggling. I'm not saying have a piece of St. Honoré cake every day, but when you are at a good French restaurant, treat yourself to a memorable dessert. You do not have to eat all of it and the pleasure of it will last.

Don't:

- Start the day with a croissant or baguette.
- Get hooked on triple crème cheeses with a hunk of French bread.
- Order French onion soup with toasted bread and cheese on top.
- Eat pâté, fatty meats, duck, and sausages.
- Have any dish prepared in cream or cheese sauces, including au gratin, hollandaise, béarnaise, and béchamel.
- Even think about trying cassoulet, a rich casserole made with beans, sausage, duck, goose, lamb, and pork. It's delicious, but the fat content of the meat is off the charts.
- Eat an entire cone of French fries.

Thai

Get ready for exotic flavor combinations in this remarkable cuisine, which is one of my favorites. A word of warning: If your server asks you how hot you want your food, be conservative. Thai chiles can make your eyes water and set off a coughing fit. Build the heat slowly or you will be sorry. I can vouch for that.

Do:

- Try *tom yum goong*, a hot-and-sour shrimp soup, which balances flavors beautifully. Talk about hitting the bliss point. This soup consists of lean meat and mushrooms simmered in broth with cilantro, lemongrass, and other seasonings. It's a caloric bargain!

- Start with summer rolls. Soft rice paper is wrapped around raw vegetables, usually carrots and sprouts, rice noodles, shrimp, and mint. Think of them like healthy egg rolls. They are light and refreshing.
- Have papaya salad, which is crispy and is served in a chile-lime dressing.
- Order satays, grilled meat skewers served with peanut dipping sauce. Go light on the sauce.
- Get acquainted with *larb*, a very spicy dish made with coarsely chopped chicken, pork, or beef. Delicious!
- Enjoy *gai pad mamuang him ma pahn*, an unforgettable cashew chicken.
- Choose *gaeng pah*, country-style curries made with water. Warning: they are spicier than coconut-based curries because there is no fat from coconut.
- Reduce your sodium intake the day you are going to eat Thai food. Fish sauce, shrimp paste, and curry paste are very high in sodium.

Don't:

- Order coconut soup—it's like eating a cream-based soup.
- Choose coconut-based curries, which are very rich.
- Eat *massaman* curry, which is like the thick versions of curry made in India. It's cooked with potatoes, crushed peanut, and coconut cream. It's too calorie intense.
- Succumb to sweet, sticky rice. It's not for you.

Spanish

The Spanish tradition of eating tapas, small plates of food, fits right in with portion control. Another plus is that the cuisine relies on fresh seafood, vegetables, and olive oil, all of which are staples in your new diet.

Do:

- Construct a meal from tapas by focusing on olives, seafood, vegetables, beans, and fresh grilled sardines and anchovies.
- Snack on fresh almonds.
- Order gazpacho, a cold tomato and pepper soup.
- Try green gazpacho, which is made from cucumber, green bell pepper, green grapes, and herbs.

- Enjoy the delicious seafood stews and fish soup, which are a good alternative to paella. No rice is involved.
- Order grilled fish and seafood.
- Have a Spanish omelet made without potatoes.
- Sample the extraordinary ham and Manchego cheese, made from sheep's milk.
- Take advantage of the wonderful citrus grown in Spain. The Spanish incorporate citrus into many of their dishes.
- Order fruit for dessert.

Don't:

- Get hooked on *pan con tomate*, grilled bread rubbed with garlic, olive oil, and tomato. Often served with Iberian ham, it is addicting.
- Eat fatty sausage—chorizo, for example—which appears in many Spanish dishes. Have just a taste, and then push the sausage aside.
- Order empanadas, the Spanish take on a Hot Pocket.
- Eat the rice and sausage in paella. Just sample both and concentrate on the seafood and chicken.
- Order *arroz con pollo*, rice with chicken. There are plenty of chicken dishes without rice.
- Inhale an entire order of flan, an egg custard served with a caramelized sugar sauce.

Indian

When you walk into an Indian restaurant, you are hit with the mouthwatering aromas of the many spices that create the distinctive flavors of Indian food, including turmeric, red chiles, cumin, cinnamon, coriander, and cardamom. Yogurt and lentils are major ingredients of the cuisine as well.

Do:

- Find out how the *papadum* are prepared before nibbling. *Papadum* are the wafer-thin disks that are brought to the table with sauces when you are seated. The ingredients are healthy: chickpeas, rice flour, black gram flour, and lentils. They are either fried or cooked with dry heat. If the *papadums* have been prepared with dry heat, nibble away. You know what to do if the *papadums* are fried.

- Have Mulligatawny or lentil soup. Mulligatawny is made with vegetables, consommé, and curry spices.
- Stick with chicken or seafood.
- Eat anything cooked tandoori style, which is oven grilled. The kebabs are delicious.
- Use *raita*, made from cucumber and yogurt, as a sauce for your tandoori.
- Choose dishes made with chickpeas or lentils, such as dal or dishes labeled *chole*.
- Enjoy veggie dishes like *aloo gobi*, which is made with cauliflower, and *sukhi bhindi*, an okra dish.

Don't:

- Start with fried appetizers, such as samosas and *pakora*.
- Eat the breads, called naan, *paratha*, or stuffed breads.
- Overdo the chutneys, which are blends of dried fruits and spices, and can be sweet.
- Pile up your plate with rice.
- Eat rich curries. They are too creamy.
- Order dishes that include *paneer*, ghee, or *malai*. *Paneer* resembles full-fat cottage cheese, ghee is clarified butter, and *malai* is a cream used to make sauces.

You are now prepared to eat at the most popular of ethnic restaurants. You have the information you need to order a meal that will not set you back. These cuisines all use herbs and spices to create the distinctive flavor profiles of each country. The guidelines for the Spice Diet apply to these exotic cuisines as well. When you want to go out or order food in from these cuisines, you are now equipped to maneuver your way around menu items that can undermine your determination to eat healthfully.

Fast Food Doesn't Have to Be a Disaster

I can assure you that it is not realistic to think you will never have fast food again. You might find yourself on line at a fast-food restaurant to order lunch for your children or grandchildren on a busy day. You just might not be able to resist the lure of the drive-thru window now and then. The good news is that demand for healthy options has grown. Most national chains have added items to their menus for the health-conscious. Just as you have to know what to order at a restaurant, you can stay on track with some advance preparation for making the right choices at a fast-food restaurant. I have compiled a list of the healthiest food you can order at the major fast-food chains. Of course, menus change all the time, but these suggestions will steer you in the right direction.

A&W:

- Three-piece Chicken Tenders (260 calories)
- Chili (190 calories)

Arby's:

- Chopped Farmhouse Salad with Roast Turkey and Light Italian Dressing (250 calories)
- Grilled Chicken Cordon Bleu Sandwich, without mayo (390 calories)
- Martha's Vineyard Salad, without dressing (277 calories)
- Santa Fe Salad with Grilled Chicken, without dressing (283 calories)

Au Bon Pain:

- Apple Cinnamon Oatmeal (280 calories)

Baja Fresh:

- 1 Grilled Wahoo Fish Taco with avocado (230 calories)

Burger King:

- Tendergrill Chicken, Apple, Cranberry, Garden Fresh Salad (380 calories)
- Tendergrill Chicken Sandwich, no mayo (350 calories)
- BK Veggie Burger, no mayo (310 calories)
- Whopper Jr., no mayo (260 calories)
- Premium Alaskan Fish Sandwich, without tartar sauce (360 calories)
- 4-piece chicken nuggets (190 calories)
- Value-sized Onion Rings (150 calories), which have fewer calories than their fries

Carl's Jr./Hardee's:

- Charbroiled BBQ Chicken Sandwich (390 calories)
- Garden Salad with low-fat balsamic vinaigrette dressing (145 calories)
- Charbroiled Chicken Salad with low-fat balsamic dressing (295 calories)
- Ordering charbroiled is the way to go at this chain. Don't order a "Thickburger," even made from turkey. They are heavy on the condiments.

Chick-fil-A:

- 8-count Grilled Chicken Nuggets (140 calories)
- Side salad (80 calories)
- Chargrilled Chicken Cool Wrap (340 calories)
- Chargrilled Chicken Sandwich (without BBQ sauce) (270 calories)
- Chargrilled Chicken Garden Salad (180 calories)
- Chick-n-Minis Breakfast (260 calories)

Chipotle:

- Cheese Quesadilla, kids size (190 calories)
- Vegetarian Burrito Bowl with black beans, fajita veggies, and vinaigrette (420 calories)
- Chicken Burrito Bowl with brown rice and pinto beans, no cheese or sour cream (500 calories)
- 3 Barbacoa Tacos on soft corn tortillas (405 calories)

Cosi:

- Spinach Florentine Breakfast Wrap (334 calories)

Culver's:

- Soups
  - Bean with Ham (160 calories)
  - Chicken Noodle (110 calories)
  - Oven Roasted Turkey Noodle (170 calories)
  - Tomato Florentine (110 calories)
  - Vegetable Beef with Barley (160 calories)

- Garden Fresco salad with raspberry vinaigrette dressing (245 calories)
- Butterburger single (390 calories)
- Beef Pot Roast Sandwich (410 calories)
- Grilled Chicken Sandwich (410 calories)

Dairy Queen:

- Grilled Chicken Garden Greens salad with Marzetti Light Italian Dressing (170 calories)

Denny's:

- Scrambled Egg Whites, Chicken Sausage, and Fruit (230 calories)

Dunkin' Donuts:

- Egg White Flatbread (280 calories)
- Egg White Veggie Wake-up Wrap (150 calories)
- Egg White Turkey Sausage Wake-up Wrap (160 calories)
- Tuna Salad Sandwich on an English Muffin (390 calories)

Five Guys:

- Veggie Sandwich (440 calories)
- Little Hamburger (440 calories)

IHOP:

- Simple and Fit Veggie Omelette (320 calories)

In-N-Out:

- Protein Style Hamburger (240 calories)
- Hamburger with onion, ketchup, mustard no spread (310 calories)

Jack in the Box:

- Four-piece Grilled Chicken Strips (250 calories)
- Side salad with low-fat balsamic vinaigrette dressing (48 calories)
- Chicken Fajita Pita, no salsa (280 calories)

Jamba Juice:

- No. 3 Berry Topper Ideal Meal 12-ounce size (300 calories) for breakfast.

KFC:

- Kentucky Grilled Chicken Whole Wing and Drumstick (170 calories)
- Green Beans (25 calories)
- KFC Honey BBQ Sandwich (280 calories)
- KFC Tender Roast Sandwich, without sauce (300 calories)
- KFC Oven Roasted Twister, without sauce (330 calories)

McDonalds's:

- Plain Hamburger (240 calories)
- Side salad with Newman's Own Low Fat Family Recipe Italian Dressing (70 calories)
- Artisan Grilled Chicken Sandwich (360 calories)
- Southwest Salad with Grilled Chicken (320 calories)
- Premium Caesar Salad with Grilled Chicken with Low-Fat Vinaigrette (190 calories)
- Grilled Snack Wrap with Honey Mustard or Chipotle BBQ sauce (260 calories)
- Egg McMuffin (300 calories)
- Fruit and Maple Oatmeal (260 calories)
- Fruit and yogurt parfait (156 calories)

Panera:

- Breakfast Power Sandwich (330)
- Smoked Turkey Breast Sandwich on Country Bread (430)
- There is a "You Pick Two" lunch menu consisting of a half sandwich and a small salad.

Papa John's:

- Garden Fresh Pizza, two medium slices (400 calories)

Pizza Hut:

- Garden Party Thin Crust Pizza, two medium slices (460 calories)

Popeyes:

- Three-piece blackened tenders (170 calories)
- Regular green beans (40 calories)

Shake Shack:

- Shack-cago Dog (315 calories)
- Single Hamburger (360 calories)
- Chicken Dog (300 calories)

Sonic:

- Corn Dog (230 calories)
- Junior Deluxe Burger (380 calories)

Starbucks:

- Spinach and Feta Wrap (290 calories)
- Protein Artisan Snack Plate (370 calories)—a good breakfast.
- Chicken & Hummus Bistro Box (380 calories)

Subway:

- 6-inch Turkey Breast Whole Wheat Sub, no cheese, add avocado (340 calories)
- Veggie Delite Salad (60 calories)
- 8 ounces Homestyle Chicken Noodle Soup (110 calories)
- Western Egg White and Cheese Muffin Melt (160 calories)
- Subway will make most of its sandwiches without bread.

Taco Bell:

- Two Fresco Soft Tacos with Shredded Chicken (280 calories)
- Fresco Chicken Burrito Supreme (340 calories)
- Fresco-style Bean Burrito Supreme (330 calories)
- Fresco-style Steak Burrito Supreme (330 calories)
- Fresco Style Zesty Chicken Border Bowl, without dressing (350 calories)

■ The Fresco menu is designed to reduce calories by replacing heavier sauces with pico de gallo. You can just get the black beans and skip the rice.

Wendy's:

■ Ultimate Chicken Grill Sandwich (370 calories)
■ Small chili (170 calories)
■ Asian Cashew Chicken Salad, full size (380 calories)
■ Garden salad with lemon garlic Caesar dressing (130 calories)

Whataburger:

■ Apple and Cranberry Salad with low fat herb vinaigrette dressing (305 calories)—you can add chicken.
■ Jr. Whataburger Cheeseburger (340 calories)
■ Small fries (270 calories)

White Castle:

■ Two Veggie Sliders (280 calories)
■ Two Original Sliders (280 calories)—the veggie sliders have less fat

Chain restaurants now have to indicate the calories in each dish, so choosing what to eat has become easier. I am sure that fast-food restaurants will continue to offer more healthy options as the demand increases.

It's important to realize that the fast-food selections I have provided don't stand up to what you can make at home, but you can allow yourself to hit that drive-thru window if you want to once in a while. You don't have to go overboard. If the food doesn't taste good to you, don't eat it all. Your taste buds are telling you something.

Surviving Holidays, Parties, and Special Occasions

From Thanksgiving to New Year's Day, the holidays can really trip you up if you are not careful. It's such a busy time with gifts to buy, meals to plan, and parties to attend or host. You are surrounded by tons of sweets, party drinks, and high-calorie foods. All the festivities can easily disrupt your goals. And it's not just the holidays. There are so many special occasions throughout the year that can weaken your resolve: Halloween parties and trick-or-treat candy, Valentine's Day chocolate and romantic meals, Easter baskets, and Memorial Day, Fourth of July, and Labor Day barbecues. And of course there are birthdays, anniversaries, showers, weddings, and graduations to celebrate. Though there always seems to be something to celebrate, food does not have be your main focus for all celebrations. This section will give you survival tactics for getting through the holidays and other parties without abandoning your new way of eating and gaining weight.

Holidays Don't Have to Trigger an Eating Extravaganza

Do you always gain a few pounds during the holidays and make a resolution to lose weight in the new year? Do you starve yourself in January to make up for overeating in the prior weeks? You have done so much to embrace healthy eating and have seen the numbers on the scale go down. Don't undermine your hard work during the holidays. Not getting sidetracked by the temptations of the season may have been difficult in the past, but these strategies will help you stay in control of what you eat:

- **Up your exercise.** The holidays are a busy time, and exercise seems to be the first thing to go. Instead, you should exercise more to compensate for all the holiday partying. Build exercise into your schedule each day, if you only go for a walk after a big meal. Don't just collapse on the sofa! Get moving.
- **Try to be consistent with healthy eating 80 percent of the time.** You might want to have a complete blowout at one meal, but that doesn't mean you have to keep it up for an entire day. You should allow yourself some flexibility. There is no reason not to enjoy your favorite holiday foods. It's all about portion control and mindful eating.
- **Stay away from holiday office goodies.** It's easy to keep going back for a tiny piece of candy or a Christmas cookie. Try to avoid even passing where the treats are left out.
- **If you receive sweets as gifts, take them to the office to share.** Or "regift" them to someone who does not know the gift-giver.

- **If you are stressed by the demands of the season, give yourself time to relax.** Whether meditating or soaking in a hot bath, find time you can spend alone in a peaceful, calming place.
- **Don't obsess about the food. Instead, plan to do fun things with your family and loved ones.** Maybe you can establish some traditions that don't involve food, like ice skating, hiking, bike riding, or skiing. Your family could attend a holiday concert or volunteer to serve holiday meals in a homeless shelter. You can get in the holiday spirit without gorging yourself. Be thankful for all you have and enjoy the people you love.
- **If you can manage it, host a party or dinner yourself.** You get to control the menu and make certain there is plenty of healthy food to eat.
- **Be vigilant about your drinking.** Allow yourself one or two glasses of wine during a meal or a party. Drink ice water or club soda with lemon or lime the rest of the time.
- **Decide what you want to splurge on.** If you can't resist the mashed potatoes and gravy, skip the pecan pie and ice cream.
- **Keep your portions small.** If everything looks great, take very small portions of each dish so you get to taste everything.
- **If you are eating from a buffet, use a small plate.** I know I often put a lot of crazy things together as I go through a buffet line. Try to construct a balanced meal, similar to what you would usually eat.
- **Slow your eating pace.** The more slowly you eat, the less food you'll consume. It takes a full twenty minutes to experience fullness. Rather than inhaling the holiday food, enjoy the company.
- **Protect yourself from bingeing on leftovers.** You can store any leftovers in small, individual portion containers. That way you won't be picking at your grandmother's turkey stuffing until it's gone.
- **If you are really worried, don't wear pants with an elastic waist or something loose-fitting to a party.** You want to be aware that you are overindulging when your clothing feels tight.
- **Finally, don't beat yourself up if you go overboard.** Get right back on track. Your next meal gives you the opportunity to make corrections and start over.

If you can get through the holidays and still manage to maintain your commitment to healthy eating, you will reinforce the good habits you have begun to establish. That's most of the battle in getting down to the weight you want to be.

How to Finesse a Cocktail Party or Cocktail Hour

Whether it's your neighbor's holiday party, an event at a business conference, an elaborate cocktail hour at a wedding, or pre-meal cocktails and finger food, navigating cocktail hour can be a dangerous course. Hors d'oeuvres look so small and harmless, but that is deceptive. Those bite-size nibbles can be extremely high in calories. It's easy to eat a full day's worth of calories by helping yourself to treats wrapped in flaky pastry and filled with cheese and crème fraîche. When you are done popping one offering after another into your mouth, you might not even feel full. Here are my suggestions for sparing yourself from cocktail party backsliding:

- **Have a healthy snack at home about an hour before leaving for the party.** An apple or a protein bar can take the edge off your hunger in a healthy way.
- **Scope out what's being served.** Walk through the party and observe what is being served on platters and at stations. When you know what the choices are, you can plan what you will eat. As you roam through the party, socialize. Greet friends, family, and business associates.
- **Delay eating anything for ten minutes.** Start with a glass of club soda or ice water. If you dive right in, you risk continuing to eat everything in sight.
- **Stand far away from the hors d'oeuvres tables and kitchen door as you can.** Focus on the people and not the food. You can make a small plate of healthy options eventually.
- **Avoid mixed drinks, which can be very caloric.** A glass of wine, champagne, prosecco, or vodka on ice are your best bets if you decide to drink. For every drink you have, have a glass of water. It will fill you up.

Dinner Parties Made Easy

When you are someone's guest for dinner, courtesy can make you uneasy about sticking to your new way of eating. After all, you don't want to be rude to your hosts. I've learned to how to be a perfect guest for dinner without abandoning my eating plan. Here's how you can do the same:

- **Find out the menu in advance if you know the host.** Many people check with guests because of food restrictions. When you know what is being served, you can plan what you will eat.
- **Offer to bring a healthy dish so that you can be sure there is something you can eat.**
- **Don't talk about how you are eating, especially if people notice that you have lost weight.** You do not want to take attention away from the food your host has gone through the trouble to prepare.
- **During cocktails, stay away from the gooey cheese and salty snacks.** By this point, you have grown to love the crunch of crudités dipped into something healthy. If the dip is sour-cream based, eat the raw vegetables. Stick with water until you are seated at the dinner table.
- **If dinner is served family style or from passed platters, you are in luck.** You can avoid all the simple carbs and serve yourself salads, vegetables, meat, poultry, or fish. Just put a drop of the sauce on the side.
- **When dinner is plated, eat the healthy food and just sample the rest.** Push what remains around a bit so as not to insult the host.
- **A friend's signature dish, such as lasagna or lobster mac and cheese, can be too delicious for you to skip.** You can help yourself to a small portion and take only a few bites.
- **Focus on enjoying the conversation with the other dinner guests rather than eating.**
- **The famous "I can't eat another bite" excuse is a way to get out of dessert.** If you can't resist, just take a few bites and enjoy them thoroughly. It should be enough to satisfy your sweet tooth. Go for the fruit if offered.
- **Remember that when other people are indulging, they want you to as well.** They can be persistent, particularly about dessert. If they don't accept that you are "stuffed," just agree to have a taste.

By following these guidelines, you can have fun instead of struggling to keep your willpower strong at occasions that are supposed to be festive.

No Need to Take a Vacation from Healthy Eating

I'm on the road a lot and have learned that I don't have to leave my healthy eating habits back at home. When you travel for pleasure or business, a little bit of planning can save you from dietary disasters. Here is what I recommend to help your eating remain consistent wherever you are:

- **Make a vow to not eat at fast-food restaurants, even if you are traveling with children.** Why eat at a familiar chain restaurant when you are taking a trip to visit someplace different and can eat locally?
- **Do some advance research about the local restaurants and those in your hotel.** There is nothing worse than having to search for a place to eat when you are hungry or jet-lagged. The concierge or person at the desk can make good suggestions, too.
- **No matter how you are traveling, you can pack your own meal.** Forget the expensive food the airlines sell you. You can carry some cut up veggies and hummus, nonfat yogurt, or a salad from home. Since people are more health conscious these days, you can usually find something to eat at an airport or train or bus terminal. If you are driving, you have no excuse!
- **Pack protein bars, nuts, and fruit for snacks while traveling to your destination.** When you arrive, carry snacks for day trips.
- **If you are early for your flight, don't just sit at the gate.** Burn some calories. Stay active and walk around the terminal.
- **Drink eight ounces of water every hour of your flight.** The recirculated air in a plane's cabin can be very dehydrating.
- **Return the key to the minibar to the check-in desk.** Pick up fresh fruit, healthy snacks, and bottled water to stock your room. The prices of the contents of a minibar are astronomical, and sometimes that giant box of M&M's will call to you in the middle of the night.
- **Don't be tempted by room service late at night, either.** Rarely does anything good come from late-night snacking. Instead, go all out and order a great breakfast to be delivered the next morning. That will get

you going for the day's activities. If your hotel offers a complimentary breakfast, close your eyes to the waffles and make healthy choices.

- **Many resorts offer workout classes and yoga.** Take advantage of them.

- **If you are traveling for business, pack your workout clothes.** In the event that the hotel doesn't have a gym, they often have an arrangement with a nearby gym. If your mission on your business trip is stressful, exercise will evaporate stress and energize you. Make sure to pack your exercise bands.

- **Most people say they never gain weight when they travel.** That might be because they are more active than when they are at home. If you are touring, you can spend a lot of time on your feet. The key is to allow yourself to try new foods on vacation. Making a conscious choice to have a treat a day is reasonable. Again, you don't have to eat it all.

Vacation is a time to restore yourself. You might choose to veg out on a beach or to have an adventure seeing new things in new places. The same guidelines for healthy eating apply wherever you are. As usual, if you observe the 80/20 rule, eating right 80 percent of the time, you will not get into eating trouble. Try that cocktail with an umbrella in it, a local dish, or a luscious dessert. With portion control in mind, sample instead of feasting. You will find that eating clean is not difficult to do wherever you are.

In this chapter, I have shared the strategies that work for me in challenging situations. Staying mindful is essential to supporting your healthy eating habits. Knowing that you do not have to be very rigid about what you eat will make it easier to follow the plan. *The Spice Diet* is not about the two D's—denial and deprivation. It's about taking control, eating delicious food, feeling blissfully satisfied, and looking and feeling better than ever. Now *that's* something worth keeping up.

AFTERWORD

Own Your Cooking Skills for Good

In these pages, I have tried to share the lessons I learned by trial and error to help you feel great and to get to a healthy weight for good. As you know, that struggle was the story of my life until not so long ago. What saved me was that I created a way to eat that fulfilled my cravings and put an end to my food addiction. My mission in writing this book was to reach as many people as I can by translating my approach to food into a practical program that really works, a plan for long-term change. I hope *The Spice Diet* is helping you to overcome your self-destructive relationship with food. As you work through Phase 1, I know that you have begun to take control of what you eat and are reaping the benefits.

I hope my book earns a place in your kitchen and that you reach for it often as you plan your meals. It all starts in the kitchen. When you are involved in the process of making the meals and snacks you eat, you begin to look at food differently. There is something magical about assembling ingredients, combining them in a harmonious way, and creating layers of flavor and textures in a single dish or an entire meal. I have filled the book with many charts and lists and tons of information, because I want to take the guesswork out of enhancing the flavor of food with spices. Enjoying the aroma of the food you are cooking and watching the ingredients transform into the final product are part of the experience. I don't mean to be too mystical—well, maybe I do—I'm a chef after all. If you love food to begin with, you will love it even more when you perform magic in the kitchen.

I expect you to find that planning and preparing your own meals becomes a high point of your day, if it hasn't happened already. The experience of cooking a meal engages all your senses in a way that ordering a meal in a restaurant, having something delivered, or getting takeout never does. The pleasure factor becomes deeper and more intense when you eat homemade food, because you have invested time and effort in the kitchen and what you have made becomes an extension of yourself.

I am eager to increase the population of what I call the Spice Nation. I want to build a community of people who care about healthy eating, who support one another in their efforts to improve their health and manage their weight. No one is more enthusiastic than a person who has been given the tools to make a big change in life and succeeded. The urge to pass the good news on is spontaneous. Citizens of the Spice Nation are advocates for the theory and practice of *The Spice Diet*.

Check out my websites, www.thespicediet.com and www.judsontodd allen.com, which are linked, and my Facebook page, www.facebook.com/ Chef-Judson-Todd-Allen-Fan-Page-120189028049907. I plan to do podcasts and cooking demonstrations and to post new recipes and tips. I invite all of you to share your experience of *The Spice Diet*—both the ups and the downs. Reading other people's stories can assure you that you are far from alone. Everyone needs someone who understands the commitment you have made, to encourage you and cheer you on as you stretch for and reach your goals. I hope we get a good conversation going on my website. I welcome you to share tips and advice, gleaned from your experience, to smooth the way for others. A special request: Don't be shy about posting recipes you love. Everyone especially welcomes a suggestion for a great new snack or dessert. When you are a cook, you enjoy changing it up and try-ing something new. The Spice Nation will generously expand your cooking repertoire.

If you find yourself in Chicago, please stop by Taste 222 and try some food at our innovative restaurant. Keep your eyes open for products that I am now developing for commercial release. You can order my Chef Blend Hot Sauce—Less Hot, More Flavor—from my website.

My wish for you is that you achieve every goal on your vision board. I hope you continue to use flavor to avoid reverting to the old days of cravings and triggers, which you have put behind you. Setbacks are to be expected now and then, but if you observe the 80/20 rule, you will be fine. Just keep on cooking *The Spice Diet* way. Preparing and eating good, fresh, healthy food is the best habit you could ever develop.

ACKNOWLEDGMENTS

I am a firm believer that people are placed in our lives for a reason and a season. I stand on the shoulders of many who have affected my story and have helped mold my ability to share with others, which has given me the powerful testimony that continues to change lives.

Family is everything to me! And though there are so many family members to name, I am thankful for the support of my parents, grandparents, brother and sisters, nephews, aunts, uncles, and cousins. I would be remiss if I did not give a special thank you to my mom, Joyce Allen, who served in every role imaginable to help bring this book to fruition.

To all of my friends, thank you for being there for me every step of this journey.

In addition to my family and friends, there are many other people whom I would like to thank:

Grand Central Publishing, you have been patient, dedicated, and supportive through this process. My phenomenal editor, Leah Miller, and her assistant, Katherine Stopa. Lisa Forde, an outstanding art director who did a brilliant job with the cover. Jimmy Franco and Amanda Pritzker, thank you for your PR and marketing genius. Thank you to Sheila Curry Oakes and Karen Murgolo for your hard work and support.

Special thanks to Steve Carlis, Hank Norman, and Rebecca Bent of 2 Market Media, LLC, for helping to make one of my dreams come true—securing a book deal for me with a top publishing house. Steve, you have delivered and continue to deliver on every promise you have made! Hank, you continue to challenge and push me to be the best both on and off camera. And Rebecca, your altruism and dedication—from helping me to test recipes to creating business opportunities—is simply amazing.

David Vigliano and Tom Flannery of AGI Vigliano Literary, thank you for being stellar literary agents and securing me a book deal with a publishing company that believes in my story and is committed to seeing my work to great success.

To my coauthor, Diane Reverand, thank you not only for understanding my story but also for helping me to tell it in the pages of *The Spice Diet*. Your hard work and dedication behind the scenes has truly been invaluable. I am beyond excited for what the near future has in store for us.

Steve Harvey, in our first year working together, you shared with me that one of your goals is to make 100 millionaires. You then looked at me and said that I would be one of those individuals. Thank you for giving me the opportunity to share my healthy, flavor-inspired cuisine with you for several years as your personal chef. You continue to help me get my message out, and I am beyond grateful for your continued support.

Gerald Washington, as president of East 112th Street Productions, the Steve Harvey World Group, and the Steve Harvey Radio Network, you invested in building my reputation as I served as Steve Harvey's personal chef. By your connecting me with 2 Market Media and others, you helped me to bring my story and recipes to the lives of others. You are a man of your word, and I appreciate your help in seeing this book to completion.

Stephen Hamilton, one of the top food photographers in the world, thank you for overseeing the most amazing photo shoot for the cover. David Raine, thank you for managing and shooting the jacket image that visually sums up the essence of *The Spice Diet*.

Tanya Burke of Beyond Pursuit, you have supported me since 2009 and have been a great friend and mentor. You have worked with me in more capacities than I can imagine, from marketing and brand director to operations and official taste tester. Your valued support has helped mold me into the individual I am, and I look forward to what the future has in store for us.

Don and Liz Thompson, CEOs of Cleveland Avenue, LLC, and the Cleveland Avenue Foundation for Education (CAFÉ) respectively, I want to thank you beyond measure for your friendship and support! You both saw and experienced my passion for food and brought me on board to help bring your vision for your food-and-beverage accelerator and restaurant to life. You have poured into me on so many levels and of course support my dreams—*The Spice Diet* being one of them. Cheers to our present and the glorious future we have ahead.

Carl Ankrum of The Media MD, you have been and continue to be a great friend who has supported my culinary journey for years. From photo shoots to videography work, you are always there when I need you.

Special thanks to Adam Zickerman, author of *Power of 10*, high-intensity fitness pioneer, and owner of the InForm Fitness gyms for bringing your brilliant expertise to health and wellness. The easy, simple, and approachable workouts you created for *The Spice Diet* are an ideal addition to my diet plan.

Nathan Carter, MD, the level of expertise you brought to *The Spice Diet* as a board-certified specialist in general and addiction psychiatry is truly invaluable. Offering my readers a perspective of food addiction from your vantage point is priceless for bringing a nice balance of information for the readers.

Kenya Thomas, MD, a friend for more than twenty years, thank you for supporting me throughout my entire journey. You know me better than most. Your expertise as a physician, food scientist, and nutritional biochemist has been a great support. Words cannot express how much you mean to me.

Ambassador Ertharin Cousin, I am inspired by your work regarding food access and nutrition on an international level. I am also all smiles that you found my food to be full of flavor and nutritious. Mission accomplished.

Steve Pemberton, vice president and chief diversity officer of Walgreens, thank you for your friendship and support. It is humbling to be able to share my expertise with such a respected company that values health and wellness.

Manika Turnbull, PhD, vice president and chief diversity officer Health Care Service Corporation, you are one of kindest and most gracious individuals. Thank you for your and your organization's support of *The Spice Diet*.

Sharone Anderson, my associate chef at Cleveland Avenue, LLC, you have been a true right hand for me and I am beyond thankful. Starting out as my intern and developing into an integral part of the Cleveland Avenue team, you have grown impressively. We share many culinary values. I appreciate your support and help through my book writing process. Your future in the culinary world is bright, so buckle up and get ready.

Leslie Anderson, senior vice president business banking, US head of treasury and payment solutions for BMO Harris Bank, you continue to support me and my dreams, and I am thankful for your sharing your network and helping me see many successes.

Heidi Barker, chief communications officer for Cleveland Avenue, LLC, your creative way with words and eye for detail are outstanding. Thank you for helping me perfect the messaging for *The Spice Diet*.

Quincy Bonds of Graphix by Dzine, your graphic design work has helped to give my brand and *The Spice Diet* a beautiful visual identity.

Kourtney Gray, PhD, as my best friend and major supporter you have been the person who does not tell me what I want to hear but what I need to hear. You have been #TeamJudson from the beginning.

John W. Lee III, as a wonderful mentor and friend, you were my first client in 2005 and served as my guinea pig as I launched my creative, healthy, and flavorful recipes. I am beyond grateful for your continued support.

To my pastor, Dr. Matthew Stevenson of All Nations Worship Assembly, thank you for pouring into me exactly what I need so that I am able to pour into the lives of others.

Kimberly Hubbard, you have been an awesome friend, supporter, and mentor to me. Thank you for introducing me to your network of influencers. Many of these relationships have lead and continue to lead to amazing opportunities for me.

Gina Ciacco, as an outstanding event coordinator you have worked with some of the top authors, publishing companies, and organizations to deliver stellar programming. Thank you for sharing your network with me to secure book signing events for me.

Megan Ford, you have supported me from day one, offering yourself and organization as a resource to help advance my career. Thank you for continuing to invest in my success.

David Clark, one of my best friends. Thank you for your support and being that friend that is just as creative as I am.

To the National Association of Health Services Executives (NAHSE), thank you for being a family to me and supporting me. It is an honor to offer a healthy cooking demonstration at our national conference every year. I am thankful that the organization has committed to helping me make *The Spice Diet* a true success.

I am honored to serve as a national board member of the American Liver Foundation (ALF) and thankful for the organization's continued support.

Nicole Pittmon of Nicole Marie Events, you are a friend with a remarkable eye for detail, design, and event management. Thank you for all your help. I look forward to having an amazing book launch event designed and coordinator by the one and only.

Darwin Brown, thank you for your overall support during the writing of *The Spice Diet*. Your writing savvy, understanding of food, and legal expertise were priceless.

Kimberly Nash, you are truly a special person in my life. Thank you for being an amazing friend and supporter.

Juan Teague, you never hesitate to help and support me, and for this I am truly thankful.

To my fraternity, Alpha Phi Alpha, and my brothers of Tau Chapter, thank you for your unwavering support and encouragement.

Sam and Donna Scott, James and Mary Bell, Linda Johnson Rice, Keith and Natasha Bevans, Arnett Faulkner, Jim and Sandy Reynolds, Megan Ford, Liz Wilson—thank you to the moon and beyond for your unwavering support, encouragement, and mentorship.

Lisa Clayborn—special thanks for your PR expertise along the book journey.

I cannot physically name the countless friends, family members, and colleagues who have helped and supported me through my journey. I love you all!

RECOMMENDED READING

As you might imagine, I have a huge collection of spice reference and spice blend books. At this point, I use spices instinctively, but when I was in school and beginning to formulate the Spice Diet, I wanted to absorb everything I could about herbs and spices. If you are as excited about cooking high-flavor food as I hope you are, you might want to read more on the subject. The first three books on the list are big reference books on spices and herbs, and the last three are small, practical books about spice blends. They are all first rate.

The Spice and Herb Bible, 3rd ed., by Ian Hemphill and Kate Hemphill (Storey Publishing, LLC, 2014).

The Spice Bible: Essential Information and More Than 250 Recipes Using Spices, Spice Mixes, and Spice Pastes by Jane Lawson (Stewart, Tabori & Chang, 2008).

The Flavor Bible: The Essential Guide to Culinary Creativity, Based on the Wisdom of America's Most Imaginative Chefs by Karen Page and Andrew Dorenburg (Little, Brown and Company, 2008).

Herb Mixtures & Spicy Blends: Ethnic Flavorings, No-Salt Blends, Marinades/ Dressings, Butters/Spreads, Dessert Mixtures, Teas/Mulling edited by Deborah L. Balmuth (Storey Publishing, LLC, 1996).

The Magic of Spice Blends: A Guide to the Art, Science, and Lore of Combining Flavors by Aliza Green (Quarry Books, 2015).

Spice Mix Recipes: Top 50 Most Delicious Dry Spice Mixes (A Seasoning Cookbook) by Julie Hatfield (CreateSpace Independent Publishing Platform, 2016).

INDEX

ABOUT THE AUTHOR

Chicago native and Food Network alum, Judson Todd Allen is the "Architect of Flavor." He is the culinary lead at Cleveland Avenue, a food and beverage accelerator, and its restaurant Taste 222. Judson also owns Healthy Infused Cuisine, LLC, which manages his brand and entrepreneurial ventures. He earned a BS in food science/human nutrition, an MBA in entrepreneurship, and a master's of public health. He also studied at Le Cordon Bleu and the Ritz in Paris.